DEALING WITH
WHAT YOU NE

DEALING WITH STATISTICS: WHAT YOU NEED TO KNOW

Reva Berman Brown and Mark Saunders

519.5
B879d

1/09

Open University Press

Open University Press
McGraw-Hill Education
McGraw-Hill House
Shoppenhangers Road
Maidenhead
Berkshire
England
SL6 2QL

email: enquiries@openup.co.uk
world wide web: www.openup.co.uk

and Two Penn Plaza, New York, NY 10121—2289, USA

First published 2008

A catalogue record of this book is available from the British Library

ISBN-13: 978-0-33-521546-1 (pb) 978-0-33-521547-8 (hb)
ISBN-10: 0-33-522117-3 (pb) 0-33-522118-1 (hb)

Library of Congress Cataloging-in-Publication Data
CIP data applied for

Typeset by Kerrypress, Luton, Bedfordshire
Printed in the UK by Bell and Bain Ltd, Glasgow

Contents

Preface

Read this bit. It will save you time because it explains the kind of book this is and, perhaps more importantly, the kind of book it isn't, which will make it easier for you to decide whether you will benefit from reading it or whether you would get more out of doing something else instead.

Right at the beginning, we want to make clear that this is not the book for you if you want to cover the world of statistics in a rigorous and exhaustive manner. The guiding principle of this book is the need to know. If you are unlikely to need a particular statistical method in order to analyse the data that you have collected for your project or dissertation, then you won't find any mention of it here.

There are enough books on statistics out there, which range from relatively simple introductions to advanced mathematical expositions. This one has a different purpose. It concentrates on what you need for success in your assignment, project or dissertation, and ignores the minor roads and byways that the person very interested in statistics would be pleased to travel.

As the textbooks (which, strictly speaking, this isn't) put it, by the end of this book, you will be able to choose and use an appropriate and effective statistical technique that will allow you to analyse your data and write about your results and findings convincingly.

In a sense, this is the book that we wish we could have used during our own studies. We both spent far too long in a fog of not understanding which statistics to use, when we should be using them and why we should be using them. As a consequence, the book concentrates on particular statistical tests and the three Ws – which test, when and why – and mainly ignores the details of how to calculate them, leaving this area for the books that not only explain the mathematics behind the techniques, but also how to use statistical software to analyse your data.

This is not the book for you if you want what any normal, self-respecting textbook currently supplies: self-check and review questions and tests, case studies, practice exercises, worked examples, activities, boxes for pauses for thought or reflection, lists of learning outcomes or a companion website. Nor will it satisfy you if you want to know all about the theory behind the statistical calculations of the methods you use.

Instead, the book is intended for you if you are undertaking a social science or business and management assignment, project or dissertation as part of an undergraduate or master's qualification. It is designed to help you choose the graphs and statistics that are suitable for your data and, having got some results from your computer, to understand what they actually tell you.

The chapters that follow set out to explain the three Ws that you need so that you can produce a successful assignment, project or dissertation. However, from now on we will just refer to any of these as a 'project' as it is less clumsy. Chapter 1 deals with why you can't avoid using statistics in analysing your data, whether this is qualitative or quantitative, and what using statistics can do for your research. Chapter 2 explains the language of statistics so that you understand what the various terms used for statistical techniques and results mean. Chapter 3 clarifies why, if you are using primary data, you need to link the creation of your questionnaire or interview to your analysis plans, and when to do this. Chapter 4 deals with using tables and charts to present your data so that you and your reader (or examiner) find them easy to understand. Chapter 5 explains the statistics used to describe data and Chapter 6 deals with the statistics used to infer differences and relationships. Finally, Chapter 7 briefly summarises what you have learned and considers what you might do next. The book provides three appendices: the first provides the types of questions and statements you are likely to use in your project, and the data types associated with them; the second discusses the main statistical software that you could use to do your statistics calculations for you, and the third provides a table of the alphabet of statistics used in this book. At the end of the book, we give you a glossary of the statistical terms that have been used throughout the book, so that you have them all in one place.

Many statistics books divide statistical tests between parametric and non-parametric tests, or they deal with the available tests in terms of their increasing rigour. The main divisions of this book are based on how you will be using statistics: displaying data, describing data and inferring differences or relationships. Explanations of terms such as parametric, non-parametric and rigour are fitted into these divisions, the term which is being explained appearing in bold.

In writing the book, it was not our intention to give you the information you need to understand the whole field of statistics. Instead, we provide you with the fundamental ideas and the most commonly used techniques that you will need to organise, and then make sense of, your data. Whilst there are no mathematical proofs of the techniques discussed, there is a discussion of the rationale for the chosen statistics.

There are very many methods that can be used to analyse your data, many of them with strange names: chi-square, Kolmogorov–Smirnov, paired *t*-test. You are quite right to feel daunted and confused about which are appropriate for your needs. Which is where this book comes in. It will deal with statistics for your project on a need-to-know basis. If a statistic is interesting, but too sophisticated for your purposes, it might sometimes be mentioned, but is otherwise ignored. What you will therefore have is an explanation and presentation of those statistical activities that are sufficient for you to deal with your data, and to come up with the answers to your questions (and to get your qualification).

A final comment

We wrote this book because we want to end the fear and anxiety about statistics that we and our students endured, and that many students still endure, and to show you that you can succeed in statistical analysis of your data. There is no doubt that learning statistics takes an investment of time and effort, but this book provides you with the means both to save some of that time and effort, and also to enjoy your analysis without fear of failure.

If, after reading this book, you can understand the statistical analysis sections of the journal articles you read, and if you have found out how to make statistics work for you, the book will have accomplished what we set out to achieve.

If you have suggestions on how to improve the book to even better meet your needs, please let us know.

Reva Berman Brown and Mark N.K. Saunders
Oxford Brookes University Business School
Wheatley, Oxford OX33 1HX

August 2007

About the authors

Reva Berman Brown BA, MA, MSc, PhD was Professor of Management Research at Oxford Brookes University, where she supported the development of faculty research capacity and skills. She published widely in business and management in areas as diverse as accounting, human resource management and medieval Jewry. Reva was author of *Doing Your Dissertation in Business and Management: The Reality of Researching and Writing* (2006), published by Sage. Prior to her career in higher education, Reva was a teacher at Hendon College of Further Education and before that at St Godric's College, London. Reva also spent a few years as a freelance journalist.

Mark N.K. Saunders BA, MSc, PGCE, PhD, Chartered FCIPD is Professor of Business Research Methods and Assistant Dean (Director of Research and Doctoral Programmes) at Oxford Brookes University. He is also a visiting professor at Newcastle Business School University of Northumbria. He currently teaches research methods to master's and doctoral students. Mark has published a number of articles on research methods, service quality, and trust and organisational justice perspectives on the management of change. He is co-author of *Research Methods for Business Students* (2007), *Strategic Human Resource Management* (2007), *Employee Relations: Understanding the Employment Relationship* (2003) and *Managing Change: A Human Resource Strategy Approach* (2000), all of which are published by Financial Times Prentice Hall. He has undertaken consultancy in the public, private and not-for-profit sectors, prior to which he was employed in local government.

Chapter 1

Why you need to use statistics in your research

This chapter explains the importance of statistics, and why you need to use statistics to analyse your data.

What is statistics?

Put simply, statistics is a range of procedures for gathering, organising, analysing and presenting quantitative data. 'Data' is the term for facts that have been obtained and subsequently recorded, and, for statisticians, 'data' usually refers to quantitative data that are numbers. Essentially therefore, statistics is a scientific approach to analysing numerical data in order to enable us to maximise our interpretation, understanding and use. This means that statistics helps us turn data into information; that is, data that have been interpreted, understood and are useful to the recipient. Put formally, for your project, statistics is the systematic collection and analysis of numerical data, in order to investigate or discover relationships among phenomena so as to explain, predict and control their occurrence. The possibility of confusion comes from the fact that not only is statistics the techniques used on quantitative data, but the same word is also used to refer to the numerical results from statistical analysis.

In very broad terms, statistics can be divided into two branches – descriptive and inferential statistics.

1. **Descriptive statistics** is concerned with quantitative data and the methods for describing them. ('Data' (facts) is the plural of 'datum' (a fact), and therefore always needs a plural verb.) This

branch of statistics is the one that you will already be familiar with because descriptive statistics are used in everyday life in areas such as government, healthcare, business, and sport.

2. **Inferential** (analytical) **statistics** makes inferences about populations (entire groups of people or firms) by analysing data gathered from samples (smaller subsets of the entire group), and deals with methods that enable a conclusion to be drawn from these data. (An inference is an assumption, supposition, deduction or possibility.) Inferential statistics starts with a **hypothesis** (a statement of, or a conjecture about, the relationship between two or more variables that you intend to study), and investigates whether the data are consistent with that hypothesis.

Because statistical processing requires mathematics, it is an area that is often approached with discomfort and anxiety, if not actual fear. Which is why this book tells you which statistics to use, why those statistics, and when to use them, and ignores the explanations (which are often expressed mathematically) of the formulae in which they tend to be articulated, though it does give advice on what you should bear in mind when planning your data collection.

One of the major problems any researcher faces is reducing complex situations or things to manageable formats in order to describe, explain or model them. This is where statistics comes in. Using appropriate statistics, you will be able to make sense of the large amount of data you have collected so that you can tell your research story coherently and with justification. Put concisely, statistics fills the crucial gap between information and knowledge.

A very brief history of statistics

The word 'statistics' derives from the modern Latin term *statisticum collegium* (council of state) and the Italian word *statista* (statesman or politician). 'Statistics' was used in 1584 for a person skilled in state affairs, having political knowledge, power or influence by Sir William Petty, a seventeenth-century polymath and statesman, used the phrase 'political arithmetic' for 'statistics'. (A book entitled *Sir William Petty, 1623–1687*, written by Lord Edmond Fitzmaurice, and published in

London in 1895, quotes Petty as saying that 'By political arithmetic, we mean the art of reasoning by figures upon things relating to government'.) By 1787, 'statistic' (in the singular), meant the science relating to the branch of political science dealing with the collection, classification and discussion of facts bearing on the condition of a state or a community.

'Statists' were specialists in those aspects of running a state which were particularly related to numbers. This encompassed the tax liabilities of the citizens as well as the state's potential for raising armies. The word 'statistics' is possibly the descendant of the word 'statist'.

By 1837, statistics had moved into many areas beyond government. Statistics, used in the plural, were (and are) defined as numerical facts (data) collected and classified in systematic ways. In current use, statistics is the area of study that aims to collect and arrange numerical data, whether relating to human affairs or to natural phenomena.

The importance of statistics

It is obvious that society can't be run effectively on the basis of hunches or trial and error, and that in business and economics much depends on the correct analysis of numerical information. Decisions based on data will provide better results than those based on intuition or gut feelings.

What applies to this wider world applies to undertaking research into the wider world. And learning to use statistics in your studies will have a wider benefit than helping you towards a qualification. Once you have mastered the language and some of the techniques in order to make sense of your investigation, you will have supplied yourself with a knowledge and understanding that will enable you to cope with the information you will encounter in your everyday life. Statistical thinking permeates all social interaction. For example, take these statements:

- 'The earlier you start thinking about the topic of your research project, the more likely it is that you will produce good work.'

- 'You will get more reliable information about that from a refereed academic journal than a newspaper.'
- 'On average, my journey to work takes 1 hour and 40 minutes.'
- 'More people are wealthier now than ten years ago.'

Or these questions:

- 'Which university should I go to?'
- 'Should I buy a new car or a second-hand one?'
- 'Should the company buy this building or just rent it?'
- 'Should we invest now or wait till the new financial year?'
- 'When should we launch our new product?'

All of these require decisions to be made, all have costs and benefits (either financial or emotional), all are based upon different amounts of data, and all involve or necessitate some kind of statistical calculation. This is where an understanding of statistics and knowledge of statistical techniques will come in handy.

Why you need to use statistics

Much of everyday life depends on making forecasts, and business can't progress without being able to audit change or plan action. In your research, you may be looking at areas such as purchasing, production, capital investment, long-term development, quality control, human resource development, recruitment and selection, marketing, credit risk assessment or financial forecasts or others.

And that is why the informed use of statistics is of direct importance to you while you are collecting your data and analysing them. If nothing else, your results and findings will be more accurate, more believable and, consequently, more useful.

Some of the reasons why you will be using statistics to analyse your data are the same reasons why you are doing the research. Ignoring the possibility that you are researching because the project or dissertation element of your qualification is compulsory, rather than because you very much want to find something out, you are likely to be researching because you want to:

- measure things;
- examine relationships;
- make predictions;
- test hypotheses;
- construct concepts and develop theories;
- explore issues;
- explain activities or attitudes;
- describe what is happening;
- present information;
- make comparisons to find similarities and differences;
- draw conclusions about populations based only on sample results.

If you didn't want to do at least one of these things, there would be no point to doing your research at all.

What statistical language actually means

Like other academic disciplines, statistics uses words in a different way than they are used in everyday language. You will find a fuller list of the words you need to understand and use in the Glossary.

Variable and constant

In everyday language, something is variable if it has a tendency to change. In statistical language, any attribute, trait or characteristic that can have more than one value is called a **variable**.

In everyday language, something that does not change is said to be constant. In statistical language, an attribute, trait or characteristic that only has one value is a **constant**. Confusingly, something may be a variable in one context and a constant in another. For example, if you are looking at the spending patterns of a number of households, the number of children (which will vary) in a particular household is a variable, because we are likely to want to know how household spending depends on the number of children. But, if you are looking at the spending patterns of households which have, say, three children, then the number of children is a constant.

Strictly speaking, in statistical language, when your variables and constants are categorical (we will discuss this more in Chapter 2), for example, eye colour or nationality, they are known as **attributes**.

Discrete and continuous

Quantitative variables are divided into 'discrete' and 'continuous'. A **discrete** variable is one that can only take certain values, which are clearly separated from one another – for instance, a sales department can have 2 or 15 or 30 people within it. It cannot, however, contain $3\frac{2}{3}$ or 48.1 people. A **continuous** variable is one that could take any value in an interval. Examples of continuous variables include body mass, height, age, weight or temperature. Where continuous variables are concerned, whatever two values you mention, it is always possible to have more values (in the interval) between them. An example of this is height – a child may be 1.21 metres tall when measured on 27th September this year, and 1.27 metres on 27 September next year. In the intervening 12 months, however, the child will have been not just 1.22 or 1.23 or 1.24 and so on up to 1.27 metres, but will have been all the measurements possible, however small they might be, between 1.21 and 1.27.

Sometimes the distinction between discrete and continuous is less clear. An example of this is a person's age, which could be discrete (the stated age at a particular time, 42 in 2007) or continuous, because there are many possible values between the age today (42 years, 7 weeks and 3 days) and the age next week (42 years, 8 weeks and 3 days).

Cardinal and ordinal

We will deal with cardinal and ordinal numbers later in Chapter 2, but here we want to highlight that a 'cardinal' in statistics is not a person with high-rank in the Roman Catholic church. **Cardinal** numbers are 1, 2, 3 and so on, and they can be added, subtracted, multiplied and divided. An **ordinal** number describes position 1st, 2nd, 3rd and so on), and they express order or ranking, and can't be added, subtracted, multiplied or divided. Most of the statistical techniques created for the analysis of quantitative are not applicable to ordinal data. It is therefore meaningless (and misleading) to use these statistical techniques on rankings.

Population and sample

In statistics, the term 'population' has a much wider meaning than in everyday language. The complete set of people or things that is of interest to you in its own right (and not because the collection may be representative of something larger) is a **population**. The number of items, known as **cases**, in such a collection is its size. For example, if you are interested in all the passengers on a particular plane in their own right and not as representatives of the passengers using the airline which owns that particular plane, then those particular plane passengers are your population.

But if you do a statistical analysis of those particular plane passengers in order to reach some conclusion about, say, (1) all plane passengers heading to that destination, or (2) all plane passengers on any route on that day and at that time, then the passengers are a sample. They are being used to indicate something about the population (1) or (2). A **sample** is therefore a smaller group of people or things selected from the complete set (the population).

It hardly goes without saying that you need to be clear about whether your data are your population or a sample. Most of statistics concerns using sample data to make statements about the population from which the sample comes.

Misuses of statistics

Statistics consists of tests used to analyse data. You have decided what your research question is, which group or groups you want to study, how those groups should be put together or divided, which variables you want to focus on, and what are the best ways to categorise and measure them. This gives you full control of your study, and you can manipulate it as you wish. Statistical tests provide you with a framework within which you can pursue your research questions. But such tests can be misused, either by accident or design, and this can result in potential misinterpretation and misrepresentation. You could, for instance, decide to:

- alter your scales to change the distribution of your data;
- ignore or remove high or low scores which you consider to be inconvenient so that your data can be presented more coherently;
- focus on certain variables and exclude others;
- present correlation (the relationship between two variables, for example, height and weight – the taller people in the sample are thinner than the shorter people) as causation (tallness results in or is a cause of thinness).

It goes without saying that, because research is based on trust, you must undertake your research in an ethical manner, and present your findings truthfully. Deliberately misusing your statistics is inexcusable and unacceptable, and if it is discovered by your supervisor or examiner, retribution will be severe.

Because you are inexperienced in research, the main errors which you might make are bias, using inappropriate tests, making improper inferences, and assuming you have causation from correlations.

Bias

In ordinary language, the term 'bias' refers simply to prejudice. It could be that when the data you are using were collected, the respondents were prejudiced in their responses. You might get this kind of thing if you are eliciting attitudes or opinions. In statistical language, **bias** refers to any systematic error resulting from the collection procedures you used. For example, in a questionnaire, if the non-respondents (those who haven't answered the questionnaire) are composed of, say, a large percentage of a higher socio-economic group, it could introduce bias (systematic error) because you would have an under-representation of that group in your study. Often the people with the strongest opinions, or those who have a greater interest in the results of the research, who may derive some benefit from the results, or who have a loyalty or allegiance to express, are more likely to respond to the questionnaire than those without those views or interests. There are procedures that can deal with non-response in questionnaires and interviews. It would benefit your research if you read up about these and included them in your research design if you are collecting data specifically for your research project (**primary data**) rather than reanalysing data that have already been collected for some other purpose (**secondary data**).

Using inappropriate tests

We'll come back to this, but here we need to warn you that one of the ways in which to misuse statistics is to use the wrong tests on your data. All statistics textbooks will tell you that non-parametric tests are to be used on nominal and ordinal variables (we'll explain these terms more fully in Chapter 2) and that parametric tests are reserved for interval and ratio variables. You will find, however, that researchers, who should know better, use parametric tests on ordinal variables. But now you know better, and you won't do that.

Improper inferences

Much of statistical reasoning involves inferences about populations from data observed in samples. The reasoning may be **inductive**, in other words, reasoning from the particular (the sample) to the general (the population). However, to avoid improper inferences, you'll need to define the population carefully and use an appropriate probability sampling technique.

Concluding causation from correlations

It is a great temptation to conclude that because two factors are correlated (co related); one of these factors caused the variations in the other. You need to be careful not to fall into this trap and not to try to draw cause-and-effect conclusions from statistical data concerning correlated factors. For example, just because sales of coal are higher when the temperature is higher does not mean these sales are caused by an increase in temperature. The real reason is that, when temperature is higher, the price of coal is reduced, resulting in more coal being purchased.

The advice about avoiding these four errors is that you should question every stage of your statistical investigation, from the design of your project, through the collection and analysis of your data, to the presentation of your findings.

Data collection

We will consider issues of primary data collection in Chapter 3 when we discuss why you need to link the creation of your questionnaire or interview to your analysis plans. It is sufficient to point out here that how you collect your primary data and how you make sense of what you have collected in order to come up with credible results are not so much connected as intertwined.

You will avoid a great deal of anxiety and anguish if you undertake the planning of your analysis at the same time as you undertake the planning of your data requirements. It will prevent a number of potential difficulties such as selecting secondary data that will not enable you to answer your questions fully or, in the case of primary data, asking the wrong questions, or asking the right questions in the wrong way, or leaving out questions you should have asked. In addition, it should help you avoid finding that you don't know how to analyse or interpret the data you have got!

Chapter 2

Understanding statistical language

This chapter explains the terms that you are going to come across when you start on your statistical journey.

Basic statistical vocabulary

Before you begin to think about the three Ws – which statistical test, when to use it, and why – you need to know the meaning of five indispensable words: population, sample, parameter, statistic and variable. Briefly, a **population** is the complete set of cases that are of interest to you; a **sample** is the smaller part you have selected from the population to examine; a **parameter** is a numerical measure that describes some characteristic of a population; a **statistic** is a numerical measure that describes some characteristic of your sample; and a **variable** is any attribute, trait or characteristic of interest that varies in different circumstances or between cases.

Variables and data

Variables are the building blocks for the construction of your analysis. Once you have the cases of your sample, as far as statistics is concerned, you are going to produce a set of numbers related to whichever of their characteristics you are interested in. Samples are made up of individual cases, and these could be people, cars, months of the year, departments of an organisation, or whatever else you are interested in researching. Naturally, you will collect data about the cases in the sample for each of your variables – for example, colour, price, employment contract and so on. And, also naturally, the data for each individual case in the sample may differ on these variables – some may be red in colour and others may be blue, some may have a price of £1.99 and others £2.59, some may be on permanent employment contracts and others on fixed-term employment contracts.

As a result, one of the things that you need to look at when you examine the cases in your sample is how they vary among themselves on those variables for which you have collected data. Such variables will enable you to distinguish between one individual person or object from another, and to place them into categories. (Categories such as 'motorcycle manufacturer' or 'gender of employee' are called nominal variables (from the Latin, *nominalis*), because names are given to the different categories that the variable can take. More of this later.)

Variables can be classified using the type of data they contain (Figure 2.1). The most basic of these classifications divides variables into two groups on the basis of whether the data relate to categories or numbers:

- **Categorical**, also termed qualitative, where the data are grouped into categories (sets) or placed in rank order.
- **Numerical**, also termed quantitative, where the data are numbers, being either counts or measures.

Statistics textbooks usually develop this classification further, offering a hierarchy of measurements. In ascending order of numerical precision, variables may be:

- **Nominal**, where the data are grouped into descriptive categories by name which, although they cannot be ranked, count the number of occurrences. Examples include gender (male, female) and department (marketing, human resources, sales, ...).
- **Ordinal**, where the relative position of each case within the data is known, giving a definite order and indicating where one case is ranked relative to another. Examples include social class (upper, middle, lower) and competition results (first, second, third, ...).

- **Interval**, where the difference between any two values in the data can be stated numerically, but not the relative difference. This is because the value zero does not represent none or nothing – or, as statisticians would say, it is not a 'true zero'. Examples include temperature in Celsius (3°C, 4.5°C, 5°C, ...) and time of day (00.34, 06.04, 19.59, ...)

- **Ratio**, where the relative difference, or ratio, between any two values in the data can be calculated. This is because the value zero represents none or nothing. Examples include number of customers (9, 10, 88, ...), height of people (1.54 metres, 2.10 metres, ...) and annual salary in euros (27,540, 38,000, ...).

Finally, data can be classified in terms of the actual values that data for a specified variable can take:

- **Discrete**, where the data can only take on certain values. Examples include number of customers and annual salary.

- **Continuous**, where the data can take on any value (sometimes, as with height of people, within a finite range). Examples include height of people and temperature.

Figure 2.1: Classification of variables by type of data

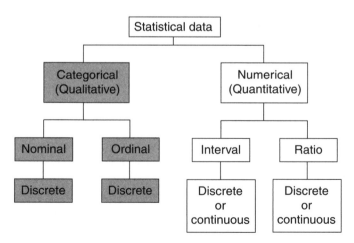

Measurement scales and variables

In statistics, nominal, ordinal, interval and ratio variables have different rules for assigning numbers that measure accurately how individuals or things differ on those variables. As the point of what you are doing is to measure your variables, you could regard measurement as the assignment of numbers to the attributes, traits or characteristics on which individual cases differ. Each of these types of data has its own **scale of measurement** and its own set of properties that define both how the numbers are assigned to them and also what you can do with those numbers in terms of statistics (Table 2.1).

Table 2.1 Measurement properties of types of data

Measurement property	Nominal	Ordinal	Interval	Ratio
		Type of data		
Can be grouped in different categories	✓	✓	✓	✓
Categories can be ranked		✓	✓	✓
Order of data values is meaningful		✓	✓	✓
Differences between data values are known and can be stated			✓	✓
Zero on the measurement scale represents total absence, showing where measurement begins				✓

Nominal scale for nominal variables

Nominal variables group data into categories, and are a type of categorical or qualitative variable (Figure 2.1). Individuals or things are assigned to categories that describe the ways in which they differ, and all people or things within the same category are assumed to be equal. On a nominal scale of measurement, codes (usually numbers) are used to represent the names (labels) of each category for a variable – for example, 1 = male and 2 = female. The coding number that you assign to each category is arbitrary, and you could choose 1 = female and 2 = male, if you prefer. The frequencies of the occurrence of the labelled categories are counted. Remember that it is not the variable's categories that are quantified – maleness and femaleness are not numerical categories, they are names or labels assigned to the variable gender. It is the frequency of the occurrence of 'male' or 'female' in the variable gender that is quantified – say, 10 males and 11 females. There is no rank order or relative size being calculated.

Ordinal scale for ordinal variables

An ordinal variable records the order or rank for an individual attribute, trait or characteristic. It is therefore possible to measure individuals in terms of position on a continuum, with one data point ranked higher or lower than another. The continuum used depends on the variable. For instance, if you ranked the educational qualifications of your respondents, a first class degree is ranked higher than a second class degree, but the difference between these (what might be called the distance between a first and a second) is not defined in your ranking. On an ordinal scale, even with rankings of first, second and third, the ranks express a 'greater than' relationship, but they don't show how much greater. We don't know whether the difference between a first class degree and a second class degree is the same as the difference between a second class degree and a third class degree. Because you are likely to have gathered much of your data in terms of ordinal variables, you need to remember that the code numbers you assign to them (say, 1 = first class degree, 2 = second class degree ...) reflect relative merit, and that the units of measurement are not equal. (We'll talk more about coding in Chapter 3.)

Interval scale for interval variables

For an interval variable, the order of the data values is known, as is the precise numeric distance between any pair of them. This means that measurements involving equal differences in the amount of the characteristic being measured are the same throughout the scale. For example, if you were measuring clocking-off times in a factory, while you know that the time difference between 4.00 pm and 5.00 pm is the same as the difference between 5.00 pm and 6.00 pm, you would never say that 3.00 pm is half as much time as 6.00, because there is no 0.00 pm which means a complete absence of time. The reason why researchers (which includes you) sometimes use rating questions (Figure 2.2) to measure attitudes on an interval measurement scale is that there is a tacit general agreement among researchers to accept the assumption that there is an equal difference between, in this example, agree, slightly agree, not sure, slightly disagree, and disagree.

Figure 2.2 A rating question

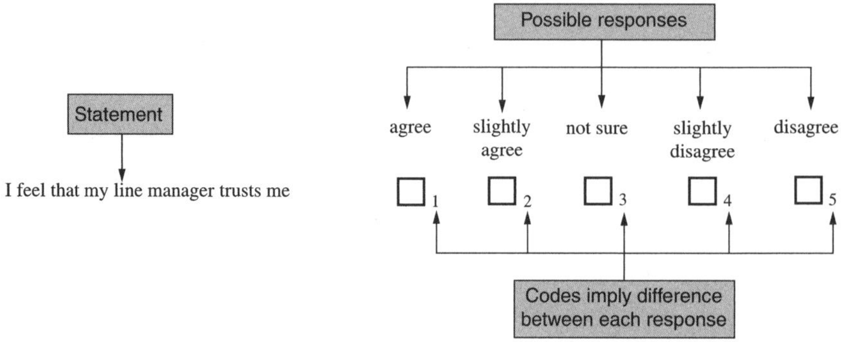

Ratio scale for ratio variables

The scale for ratio variables has a **true zero** point and equal units of measurement. This means that zero not only indicates the absence of the thing being measured (say, in terms of weight, no weight at all), but also shows the point where measurement begins. The equal units of measurement provide consistent meaning from one situation to the next and across different parts of the scale. This makes it possible to say not only that, in Dublin, €10,000,000 is twice as much as €5,000,000, but that €10,000,000 is twice as much as €5,000,000 wherever in the world currency is measured in euros.

Relationships between variables

When using statistics to analyse your data, as well as describing and presenting what you have found out about individual variables you will need to talk about differences between variables and relationships between variables. When talking about such analyses, statistics books classify variables in terms of how you use them in relation to other variables in your analysis. Whilst we talk about this more in Chapter 6, here it is worth considering two terms:

- **Independent** variable, which is the variable manipulated (altered or changed) to find out its effect on another variable. This is usually represented by the lower-case letter x.

- **Dependent** variable, which, as the focus of most statistical analysis, is the variable that is measured in response to the manipulation of the independent variable. This is usually represented by the lower-case letter y.

For example, in a study of mobile phone use we might make the assumption that the number of calls made and the average length of time spent on each call were both dependent upon the age of the mobile phone user. Number of calls and average length of time spent on each call would be our dependent variables while, age of mobile phone user would be our independent variable.

As you might expect, there are other labels given to variables when talking about relationships – for instance, exploratory, predictive, and dummy variables – but as you are unlikely to need to use them for your analysis, we mention them and pass on. You will find them in a more mathematical statistics textbook if it turns out that you do need them.

Analysing data

A statistic is a number that summarises some characteristic about a collection of data. Every **data set** (collection of data) tells a story, and if you use statistics appropriately, the data set will tell your story well and clearly. It is therefore important that you make good decisions about how to analyse the data you have collected for your research.

Whether you have categorical or numerical data, you are going to want to know about your data and answer your questions. And, sensibly, you will begin by analysing what you have collected to:

- make sense of the data you have gathered;
- provide you with information that is easy to understand;
- clarify what might be complicated;
- discover relationships and differences;
- make points clearly and concisely.

To make sense of your data, we suggest you start by presenting them as tables and graphs. Both tables and graphs will help you summarise your data, making it easier to understand. Subsequently, you can use statistics to describe individual variables, clarifying what might seem complicated, and to discover whether there are differences or relationships between variables.

Presenting data

Data presentation refers to the use of tables and graphs to illustrate your data. While you will find more information about this in Chapter 4, here is an initial taster of what is to come. Tables are a good way to summarise categorical information. For example, suppose you have categorical data about the age and gender of people in the sales department of the firm or firms you are interested in. You might create a table with column headings such as Age, Number of males, Percentage of males, Number of females, Percentage of females, Number of employees, Percentage of employees; see Table 2.2. (This is a somewhat clumsy table, but it does illustrate what you can do, and how it can save you a great many words of description.) What is worth drawing your attention to is that while age is strictly a numerical (ratio) variable, in this instance, because the age has been recoded into ordered categories (of age range), it has been presented as categorical (ordinal) data.

This kind of table can present a great deal of information – for instance, you can see whether or not men in a certain age category outnumber women in the same age group, or which age group has the smallest proportion of men.

Because you have collected the data on the number of men and women in your data set, you can calculate the percentages of men and women in the categories you require. But it doesn't work the

Table 2.2   Annotated table extract showing sales department employees by age and gender table

Numerical variable: age					Categorical variable: gender	

Sales department employees by age and gender

Age	Males		Females		All employees	
	Number	Percent	Number	Percent	Number	Percent
under 18	4	7.4	6	15.8	10	10.9
18–29	14	25.9	7	18.4	21	22.8
30–39	15	27.8	9	23.7	24	26.1

Recoded into ordered categories and presented as ordinal data

Percentages calculated separately for columns

other way around – you can't work out the number of people from percentages. For instance, if you know how many women there are in the sales department, you can work out the percentage of how many of the women are over 50. But if you were given the statistic that 10% of the women in the sales department are over 50, you have no way to work out how many women there are in the department.

You can also present your data using graphs. These also provide a simple and effective way to explore and understand your data. As you will see in Chapter 4, graphs can be used to show the values of a single variable or, as in Figure 2.3, the relationship between two variables. The precise graph you use depends upon the type of data variables and what you are trying to show. Figure 2.3, a multiple bar chart, has been drawn to compare the number of sales department employees (ratio) in each age group (ordinal, but recoded from the ratio data of individual employees' ages) between genders (nominal). Within this multiple bar chart, placing the male and female bars for each age group next to each other makes comparisons between genders easy.

Describing data

Categorical data are concerned with characteristics of cases, such as an individual's name, gender, colour (say, of eyes, hair, car or socks) or opinion about some issue (which may be given as an answer in an

Figure 2.3 Annotated multiple bar chart showing sales department employees by age and gender

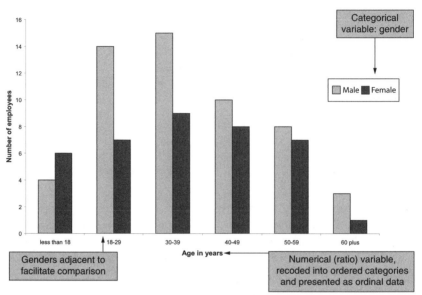

interview or questionnaire in terms of categories such as: agree, have no opinion, disagree, or better, stay the same, worse). In the main, categorical data tend to be described using percentages. To calculate a percentage is easy:

1. Take the number of cases in a certain category.
2. Divide this by the total number of cases.
3. Multiply the result by 100.

With numerical data, the variables that you are concerned with include measurements and counts such as weight, height, age, or income, and so on, and these are obviously expressed as numbers. Because these data have numerical meaning, you can describe them in more ways than you can describe categorical data. What is comforting is that these descriptive statistics can often be done without needing complicated statistical software – your fingers and some mental arithmetic, or a calculator, will do just as well. As you will see in Chapter 5, descriptive statistics allow you to describe where the centre is; that is, where the middle point of the data is, or what a typical value might be, and how much the data differ from (are dispersed) around this middle value. And, clearly, the method that you choose to find the centre of a data set influences the conclusions that you can draw about your data.

Inferring differences and relationships

One way you can begin to look for relationships between variables in your categorical data is by creating a cross-tabulation (often referred to as a 'crosstab' by statistical software). This enables you to summarise information about two categorical variables at the same time – for instance, gender and age (Table 2.2). Using statistical software, cross-tabulations can also give you the percentage of individuals in each combination of categories that you have chosen – for instance, where gender and age are concerned, the percentage of women who are aged 20–29. Cross-tabulations present data in tables (see Chapter 4). The usefulness of cross-tabulations is that you can move on from them to conduct statistical tests to find out whether there is a link between the two variables of concern – in formal language, infer whether there is a significant relationship between the two identified variables or if the difference, for example in the number of males and females within each age group, is significant. As we have already noted, the statistical tests you might use to do this are called inferential statistics because they allow you to draw conclusions or inferences about a population on the basis of the data in your sample. We will discuss these in Chapter 6.

Chapter 3

Linking data collection with analysis

This chapter considers linking the creation of your questionnaire or interview to your analysis plans, and explains why you should do so. However, if you are using secondary data then you should still read this chapter as it will be helpful in understanding the relationship between how the data you are using were originally collected and the analysis you intend to undertake.

Matters of meaning

Before we begin to discuss linking your data collection instrument or instruments to your analysis, a small reminder that, in general, your research is going move from the descriptive, where you accurately show the people, events and situations that are the objects of your research, to the interpretative, where you suggest meanings that go beyond just description.

The underlying question of all research is "What does it mean?" 'Meaning' can denote four things:

- explaining why things happen as they do (causation);
- estimating future outcomes (prediction);
- drawing comparisons;
- evaluating.

The interpretation of meaning can focus on:

- function (what role did different variables play?);

- process (what was the sequence of events?);
- person (what were the individual's or group's motives and emotional reactions?);
- comparison (what were the differences or relationships between individuals or groups?);
- evaluation (how effective were the behaviours or procedures under investigation?);
- consequences (what followed an event or incident?).

Designing your research

There is a very irritating proverb (irritating because it is true) – a stitch in time saves nine. And we've all been there. Ignore a small snag in an item of clothing that would have taken a couple of stitches to repair, and it grows into a genuine tear that needs much more attention, and takes up far more time to deal with than if you'd given it those few minutes in the first place.

The same thing applies to designing your research, including both selecting your sample and creating your data collection instrument. For example if, while you are writing the questions and statements that you are using to collect data, you give thought to how you intend to analyse the responses, and make a note of this, you will find that you have saved yourself hours of time and a great deal of effort when it comes to analysis.

If you wait until the analysis stage to decide what to do, you are likely to find that some data that you need won't have been collected and some will have been collected in the wrong form that makes it extremely difficult to find an appropriate statistical test to analyse them.

Paying attention to the population and sample

Any good research methods textbook will deal with the issues of the population and the sample thoroughly and well. What we present for you below is general advice to bear in mind when you are thinking about collecting as well as when you are analysing your data.

As we've mentioned before, the population of your research is the complete set of cases, which is the focus of attention in your research. The sample is the smaller group of cases which have been selected in some way from the population. Your intention is to draw conclusions about the sample from which you can generalise (make inferences) in differing degrees of strength and accuracy about the rest of the population from which you chose your sample.

Selecting the sample

The conclusions that can be validly drawn, and the inferences that can be validly made, from your sample depend on both the population you have sampled, and the procedures you used for generating the sample.

There is no need here for us to go into the details of sampling. We assume that you will already have a research methods textbook that you can consult, and that will cover the various types of sampling available to you – probability and non-probability.

What we do need to mention is that your sample is crucial for the success or failure of your research, and that therefore you will be doing yourself a great disservice if you don't take great care about selecting the right sample for your research. You don't want to contemplate the horror and distress of finding, when you do start your analysis, that you have chosen the wrong sample or that you don't have enough interviewees or questionnaire respondents to enable you to produce robust and believable findings.

Sample size

Because any statistical method requires a minimum size of sample to have a reasonable likelihood of discovering what you wish to find out, the decisions that you make about the size of your sample will have repercussions through all the research you undertake. There are statistical procedures that can be used to decide on the size of your sample, and you will find information about the sample sizes necessary for a particular statistical procedure in any book that provides a more detailed account of statistics, and how to use statistical techniques.

Unfortunately, there is no precise way to calculate the best size for a sample. The rule of thumb is that you need a sample of at least 30 respondents for most statistical tests. We don't need to point out the obvious – that the larger the size of the sample, the more accurate the information on the population is likely to be. Above a certain size (depending on the test you intend to carry out, and which therefore is difficult to define), you might find that it isn't worth the cost in time and money to get what ends up being a small amount of extra information about your population. The advice we can give you is to use your common sense, together with any information you already have in your research methods text, and with your supervisor's advice, to estimate an appropriate sample size.

Think about things such as how much specialist information you will need to get results that will be a true representation of what you have set out to discover, and how likely it is that the sample is representative of the population.

Choosing the sample

Samples can be classified into two distinct groups based on whether it is possible to obtain a **sampling frame** that is a complete list of the total population (Figure 3.1).

- **Probability** or **representative samples** are where each case in the population has a known probability or likelihood of being selected for the sample. Selected at random, they are used if you are intending to make statistical inferences about your population. To do this you need a suitable sampling frame. Your research methods textbook will explain the different probability samples available to you, for example, simple random, systematic random, stratified random and cluster.

- **Non-probability** or **non-random** samples are where the probability of each case being selected from the total population is not known as you do not have a sampling frame. This means you will not be able to make statistical inferences about a population from your sample as it will have been selected in a non-random manner. In an attempt to overcome this where the sampling frame is not known, quantitative researchers often use a quota sample. A

quota sample is based on the idea that your sample will represent a population if the variability for certain known 'quota' variables, often age and gender, are the same in the sample as the population. For qualitative research, the non-probability sample that you select is likely to be much smaller than a probability sample, but the data collected are likely to be more detailed than in the case of a probability sample. Your research methods textbook will explain the different non-probability samples available to you, for example, purposive, snowball, self-selection and convenience.

Figure 3.1 Types of sample

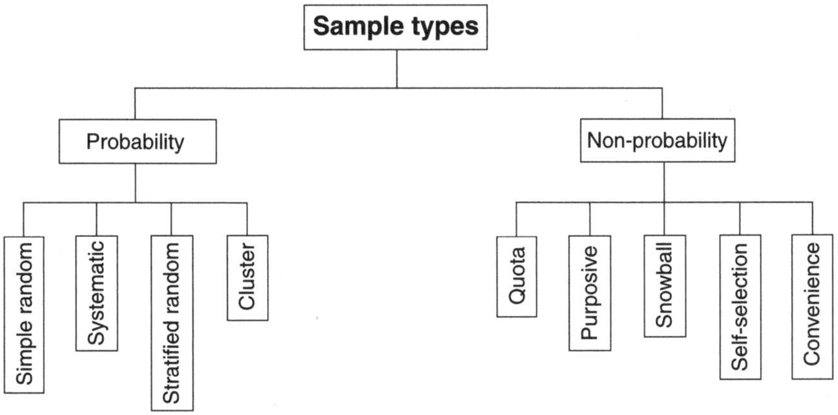

Populations

It is sometimes possible to collect data from every member of the population, if this is small enough. This is a liberation for you, because it removes the necessity to think about sampling issues and the potential difficulties of representativeness, validity, reliability, generalisability, and bias.

When you are collecting data from a population, the term used is **conducting a census**, which means collecting data from every case in the population about whatever it is you need to find out. It isn't easy, but it might be worthwhile to think about whether you could use every case rather than a sample of cases for your project.

Preparing data for analysis

Assuming that you have selected the right sample and the right data collection method and data collecting 'tool' or 'instrument' (formal language for 'interview' or 'questionnaire'), then once you have collected all the data that you need for your project, you will need to prepare your data for analysis. Once you have done this you will be able to solve your research problem or answer your research question. (Sometimes this is easier said than done, but it is rarely impossible to do.)

Checking the raw data

The first thing you will do, once you have done your data collection, is to check your raw data. What you are aiming to do by checking is to:

- make sure that the data are accurate, complete, and consistent with the intent of the questions asked, statements and other information;

- make sure that the data from pre-coded questions have been coded correctly using the codes decided upon;

- make sure the coding schedule developed for questions that were not pre-coded is appropriate and has been applied correctly.

Subsequently, once you have typed in (entered) the data into the statistical software, you will need to check that this has been done correctly before starting your analysis.

If you find a response that is inconsistent or illogical (a respondent aged 18 with 30 children!), missing, or has been coded incorrectly, there are three main things you can do about it:

- Check the raw data to see if it was a data entry error and, if it was, correct it.

- If the data collection was not anonymous, it might be possible to go back and ask for clarification.

- Accept that it is incorrect information, code it as 'missing data', 'non-response' or 'unknown', and ignore it in subsequent analyses.

One of the easiest ways to check your data once you have entered it is to create frequency tables for each variable (Chapter 4). We have found this really helpful in discovering data that have been miscoded using illegitimate codes, that is ones which do not exist in your coding scheme.

A word of advice – take care not to destroy, erase or make illegible the original questionnaires or interview notes. Use a variable as an identifier to link the questionnaire or notes for each case to the data you enter into the statistical software, and then put the transcripts or questionnaires aside and keep them safe, until your project has been assessed and the mark awarded. You never know, if you don't do as well as you expected or hoped, you might be given the opportunity to improve your project or dissertation, if it isn't quite up to scratch, and then you will be very glad that you are able to return to these original documents and consult them.

Data coding

This is where your stitch in time comes in. At the same time as you create the questionnaire or interview schedule, insert the codes against each question or, for open questions, make a note of the coding schedule you intend to use. You can keep the coding on the master copy and not put it on the documents that you will use for the interviews, or send to questionnaire respondents, but we can't impress on you strongly enough the advantage you will have given yourself if you pre-code questions wherever possible at the same time as you design and create the questionnaire or interview schedule.

Coding is the assigning of numbers or other characters to answers so that the responses can be grouped into classes or categories. It may be that putting your data into these categories sacrifices some data detail, but it will do wonders for your analysis. Good coding will help you to group, say, several hundred replies into the few categories that you need in order to analyse your data. The formal language is that you are using categories and employing categorisation: **catego-**

ries are the partitioned subsets of your data variable, and **categorisation** is the process of using rules (defined by you) to partition your data into these subsets.

Codes are normally numeric, although they can be alphabetical or alphanumeric. Take the example of gender, where you have the categories 'male' and 'female'. The coding would be **numeric** if you code this as '1' for male and '2' for female (or as '0' for male and '1' for female, or any other two numbers that you prefer). It would be **alphabetical** if you code male as 'M' and female as 'F', and **alphanumeric** if you used a combination of letters and numbers such as 'M2' for male and 'F2' for female.

Rules underlying coding

When you are designing your coding, you will have in mind the categories and potential categories that you wish to analyse. Often these will be based on existing categories, such as those devised for government surveys, with which you might want to compare your own data. It is common sense to add that to guide you in the coding of your data into initial categories for analysis, and for effective and successful results, the coding of your categories should be:

- appropriate to the research problem and purpose;
- exhaustive;
- mutually exclusive;
- derived from one classification principle.

Appropriate to the research problem and purpose

Your categories must provide the best partitioning of data for testing and uncovering what you wish to find out – for instance, if specific age groupings of your respondents or their income or departmental position are important to your research, then, when you are designing your data collection tool, you must choose those groupings that will best provide you with exactly the information that you want, which will then enable you to code in the best way to discover what you wish to know. For example, it would be unhelpful to your analysis if you have asked for, say, age in the five-year bands 0–4, 5–9, 10–14, 15–19,…, when you need the actual age in years for your analysis purposes, or alternatively, the secondary data with which you wish to compare your findings are only available in year bands 0–5, 6–10, 11–15, 16–20,…. This is obviously why, when designing the data collection document, considering the potential categories and designing the coding for them is the best thing you can do to help yourself get good results.

Exhaustive

It is easy to say, and not all that easy to do – you need to ask all that you wish to know. When you have used multiple-choice questions, you need to be careful to provide a full list of alternatives. Using the category of 'other, please describe' (Figure 3.2) at the end of your list of alternatives can be helpful, and can also be damaging. A large number of 'other' responses show that your list (category set) is too limited. As a result, you won't have gathered the full range of information that you want, and any answer that you haven't actually specified in your multiple-choice questions is likely to be under-represented, because you have no control over whether or not your respondents decide to put the item in the 'other' space.

Figure 3.2   Annotated pre-coded question using 'other'

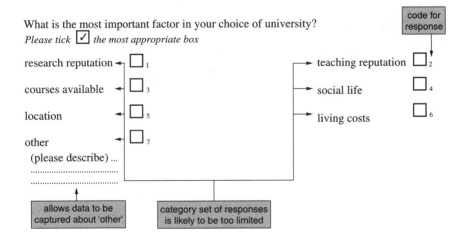

Mutually exclusive

Mutually exclusive categories mean that a specific answer can be placed in only one category. For instance, say you have asked your respondents to place themselves in an occupational type. You intend that they should choose only one in your list, perhaps '1' = professional, '2' = managerial and '3' = administrative. It could be, however, that a respondent who is head of the accounting department considers him or herself as both a professional and a manager. Your coding scheme can't cope if this person therefore ticks both boxes, because you have set up your codes to allow only one entry in this category. A way to prevent this kind of thing is to make sure that you define what you mean by professional, managerial, and administrative, so that the respondent understands exactly what you mean, and will choose only one, as you have requested.

Derived from one classification principle

What this means is that all the categories for a variable are defined in terms of one concept. For instance, if you had added to your list of occupation types '4' = unemployed, then you would have two concepts in this category: professional, managerial and clerical are occupational types, but unemployed is current occupational status. The latter has nothing to do with the occupational type, because a person can be an unemployed professional, unemployed manager, or unemployed administrator, but unemployment is not a type of occupation. Logically, then, if a category set uses more than one dimension, it can't be mutually exclusive.

Using a code book

You will find it very useful to create a coding scheme or **code book**. This should contain the question number, variable name, variable label, code and associated label of the code for the response options. Table 3.2 shows an extract from a code book.

Table 3.2   Extract from a code book

Question	Variable name	Variable label	Code and value label
	ID	Case identifier	4-digit number given to questionnaire
1	BIRTH	Year of birth	Birth year (2-digits), e.g. 1 9 _ _ blank = missing
2	GENDER	Gender	1= male 2 = female blank = missing
3	CHOICE	Most important factor in your choice of university	1 = location 2 = social life 3 = courses available 4 = teaching reputation 5 = research reputation 6 = living costs 7 = other blank = missing

Obviously, if you have a robust coding scheme, it will be easy to enter your data into the statistical software that you use.

And another thing – good research requires that when you think that your data collection instrument is as good as you can get it, you do a pilot study. But it isn't enough just to ask some people to fill in your questionnaire and comment on it or do a few structured interviews. An essential part of piloting is to analyse the pilot responses – and you will need a code book in order to do that. Not only is it possible (and even likely) that the pilot collection of data will show you aspects of your interview or survey that need to be adjusted and corrected, but it may also show you where your coding scheme needs to be corrected before you collect the data for your final study, or even that you might need to rethink the statistical tests you aim to use.

Coding closed questions

The questions in your questionnaire or interview that can be pre-coded are the **closed questions** (Figure 3.2), where the questionnaire respondent or interviewer ticks a box or circles a number next to a possible answer you have already provided, in order to record their reply directly. Often it is sensible to use coding schemes that have already been developed by someone else in your research. This allows you to make comparisons with your data.

Coding open-ended questions

Clearly, closed questions are easier to code, record, measure, and analyse. But there are situations where you are unable to predict the response categories in advance. You may be exploring areas where you are looking at sensitive behaviour, or you may want to encourage natural modes of expression. **Open questions** often require narrative responses (Figure 3.3), and the trouble is that analysing large volumes of responses to open-ended questions can be a nightmare. For these questions you are going to need to create a coding scheme after the data have been collected.

Figure 3.3 An open question

Please list up to three things you like about this hotel.

1..
2..
3..

To create a coding scheme for an open question you need to:

  (i)   decide on the level of detail you require for your analysis;
 (ii)   read through the responses and establish broad categories;
(iii)   divide the broad categories into more specific sub-categories;
 (iv)   allocate codes to the most detailed sub-categories;
  (v)   note the responses for each code in your code book.

Table 3.3 Annotated extract of hierarchial coding scheme developed from responses to the open question in Figure 3.3

Question	Variable name	Variable label	Code and value label	
18	LIKE1	Thing likes about hotel (first)	100	Room
			110	Bed
			111	Comfort
	LIKE2	Thing likes about hotel (second)	112	Size
			113	Proper sheets
			120	Mini bar
	LIKE3	Thing likes about hotel (third)	121	Selection
			122	Free
			130	Ensuite
			200	Location
This question results in 3 variables each coded the same way		Code numbers reflect hierarchy	201	Central
			202	Convenient
			300	Facilities
			301	Restaurant
			321	Swimming pool
			322	Gym

Responses divided into categories

Coding questions and creating scales

Rating questions (Figure 2.2) are often used if you are interested in strength of feeling or in opinions. They are often combined to create a numerical measure for a concept such as employee stress, service quality or customer satisfaction. Each question is called a scale item and the overall scale score is created by adding the scores (codes) for each of the questions (scale items) that together make up the scale. The most straightforward and the easiest to use type of scale item is the Likert-style rating scale. This asks respondents to indicate their strength of agreement or disagreement with a given statement, by circling the appropriate number, or ticking the appropriate box, generally on a five- or seven-point range (Figure 2.2). Responses are then coded, generally from 1 = strongly agree through to 5 or 7 = strongly disagree.

Over the years literally thousands of scales have been developed, details of which are often given in research 'handbooks' and research articles. Because of this, it is often sensible to use an existing scale, subject to copyright constraints, rather than invent your own.

Coding 'don't know' or 'no opinion' responses

In your coding, you may need to take account of the fact that your respondents may wish to respond with a 'don't know' or 'no opinion' answer, and so supply this category. To minimise the potential of having a large number of 'don't know' responses, you will need to be careful about what questions you ask and how you ask them.

A word of warning, however, on an after-coding issue – when it comes to analysing these 'don't know' or 'no opinion' responses, you will have decisions to make. No matter how careful you have been, what you can't avoid is a situation where the respondent genuinely doesn't know the answer. The difficulty comes when you suspect that the 'don't know' response really means 'I don't understand the question' or 'I don't want to answer the question', or 'I find this so trivial or unimportant, I can't be bothered to think about it' or 'I don't want to do the work you are asking for (say, calculate the number of times something has happened in the past week or rank items in order of importance) to provide the information you want'.

While you are collecting the responses during semi-structured interviews, you, as the interviewer, have the opportunity to rephrase the question or to reassure the interviewee, and thus to coax a response, but with a questionnaire, there is nothing you can do to encourage a respondent not to go down the 'don't know' route.

There are, however, two ways to deal with 'don't know' responses when it comes to analysing them. If you are using a questionnaire and have given a question or statement a 'don't know' alternative, along with the 'yes' and 'no' alternatives, you should analyse the three categories. However, if you are collecting responses using semi-structured interviews and are certain the respondent does know and is refusing to answer, so that their 'don't know' is really a disguised deliberate avoidance, or indicates a reluctance to reply, then you could make an additional reporting category for such refusals and let your reader make the decision as to the relevance of these refusals to your overall results.

Data entry

Another thing to bear in mind when designing your own data collection instrument is how you intend to enter your data. In general, if you use statistical software, you are likely to have to use manual keyboard entry. If you have access to a computer image scanner, you could use optical character recognition programs to transfer printed text into computer files in order to edit and use it without retyping. Even better, if you have access to optical mark recognition (OMR) software, you could process your interview transcript or questionnaire this way. OMR is faster than manual keying, reduces input error, makes viewing the data easy, and provides charts and reports. Increasingly questionnaires are administered using the Internet or an organisation's intranet. Online questionnaire software usually automatically captures the data as each response is typed, saving it to a data file. However, they can only be used where respondents have access to the Internet or an organisation's intranet.

Moving on to data analysis

Because you will get only one chance at collecting any primary data you need, it is vital that your data collecting tool is the best that you can construct to answer your research questions. When it comes to coding, we suggest you go for the belt-and-braces method, and use the following two-stage method when designing the questionnaire or interview schedule:

1. Create a master document, in which you note down for each question or statement the bit of literature or theory that it is connected with or refers to. This makes it clear why you are asking that question and collecting the data. It is also a great help when writing up the findings, as you know which finding is connected to which theory or publication that is relevant to the research.

2. Create a code book (see Tables 3.2 and 3.3) in which the codes for each question and the reasons why those codes were chosen are noted. This will enable the data from the responses to be entered more easily and you to justify your choices of codes. These notes should not be made on the questionnaire or interview schedule and will not be seen by respondents.

Final comments

The more careful you are about linking data collection with analysis, the easier it will be to undertake your analysis, to understand what the data are telling you, to draw interesting and valuable conclusions from your findings, and, therefore, write your project report.

However, before we move on to talk about presenting and analysing data, two warnings:

- Always check the data have been entered correctly before starting your analysis. It is far easier to correct data before you start your analysis, rather than having to both correct your data and redo your analysis!

- When you start your analysis be careful that you don't make the common mistake of analysing the codes that you have selected for your nominal variables (e.g. gender, department) as numbers. We have on numerous occasions seen project reports where gender was coded male 1 for males and 2 for females, which talk about an average gender of 1.6! This is why we have insisted that you always understand what types of data your variables contain before you use any statistics.

Chapter 4

Presenting data

This chapter shows which tables and graphs to use to present your statistical data.

The main reasons why you should be using tables and graphs to display your data are:

- (in the early stages of statistical analysis) to explore and to understand the data;
- (when preparing a report or a presentation) to make your points clearly.

Tables and graphs will enable you to describe, compare and contrast variables, show relationships between variables, and present in a 'picture' what would take a great many words to describe. As, in general, categorical and numerical data (Figure 2.1) use different tables and graphs, we have structured this chapter to reflect this.

Presenting categorical data using tables

Tables present information in rows and columns, and should be used when you want to summarise information so that specific values can be grasped quickly and easily. Besides 'normal' tables that don't require any calculations other than percentages, there are others which produce the results of statistical tests in a comprehensible and concise way.

Frequency tables

A **frequency table** or **frequency distribution** summarises the number of cases in each category for a variable. This table is very helpful when you are starting out to examine your data. It gives the total number (and, if calculated, the percentage) of times each category or value occurs (the **frequency** with which it occurs). This is often represented by statisticians by the lower-case letter f, whilst the lower-case letter x is used to represent all the individual data values of a variable.

Table 4.1, created using the statistical software SPSS, shows responses to the statement 'The event was value for money'.

The table presents the frequencies as a number (Frequency), as a percentage of both those respondents who returned the questionnaire (Percent) and of those who answered the question (Valid Percent). The cumulative percentage has also been calculated and presented. Often in tables, the letter n is used as a column heading to signify the total. Strictly speaking, a lower-case n should be used to signify the total for a sample, whereas an upper-case N should be used to signify the total for a population.

Table 4.1 Annotated frequency table

Categories	Number of respondents	Percentage returning the questionnaire	Percentage answering the question

The event was value for money

		Frequency	Percent	Valid Percent	Cumulative Percent
Valid	Strongly Disagree	6	.9	.9	.9
	Disagree	23	3.3	3.6	4.5
	Agree	395	57.4	61.8	66.4
	Strongly Agree	215	31.3	33.6	100.0
	Total	639	92.9	100.0	
Missing	System	49	7.1		
Total		688	100.0		

Number of respondents for whom data are missing for this question	Percentage of respondents for whom data are missing for this question

Cross-tabulations

Cross-tabulations or cross-classification tables are used when you need to present a table that summarises more than one variable at the same time. In these two-way tables, the categories of one of the variables form the rows and the categories of the other variable form the columns. When you interpret your cross-tabulation, remember that while the one variable doesn't cause the other, the table does show the relationship between the two variables. Table 4.2, created using the spreadsheet Excel, shows the relationship between responses to the statement 'The event was value for money' and respondents' age groups.

Table 4.2 Annotated cross-tabulation

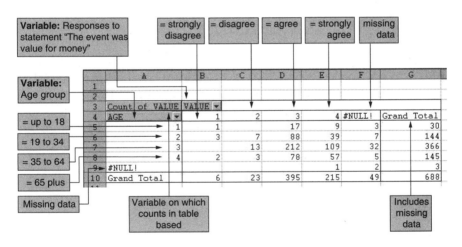

Before Table 4.2 could be included in a report or presentation, it would be important to use more easily understandable names for each of the variables, replace the codes for each variable with their labels, add a title and state the source of the data the table contains (Table 4.3). As a rule of thumb, your table should be clear enough to allow it to be understood without having to read any of your text!

Table 4.3 Annotated cross-tabulation for a report

Title clear and in bold

Columns (and rows) in sensible sequence

Column (and row) headings clear

Table 4.2

Age by perception of event's value for money

Units stated

Row (and column) headings in bold

Age (years)	Response to "The event was value for money"				
	strongly disagree	disagree	agree	strongly agree	Total (=100%)
up to 18	3.7	0	63.0	33.3	27
19 to 34	2.2	5.1	64.2	28.5	137
35 to 64	0	3.9	63.5	32.6	334
65 and over	1.4	2.1	55.7	40.7	140
All ages	0.9	3.6	61.9	33.5	638

Notes: 50 respondents did not provide data for this table; percentages may not sum to 100 due to rounding errors.

Notes explain irregularities

Source: Audience Survey, 6 April 2008

Source of data stated

Presenting categorical data using graphs

There are a wide range of graphs available. However, only some of these are suitable for presenting categorical data. Those most frequently used are summarised in Table 4.4 along with when to use them. Those shaded in Table 4.4 are the ones you are most likely to use. You will probably have little use for those graphs not shaded.

Table 4.4 Graphs for presenting categorical data and when to use them

Graph	Use when you want to present data to
Bar chart	show frequency of occurrence and emphasise highest and lowest categories for one variable (frequencies are normally displayed vertically and categories horizontally) show the trend for one variable over time (frequencies are normally displayed vertically and discrete time periods horizontally)

Pie chart	emphasise proportions in each category for one variable
Multiple bar chart	compare frequency of occurrence for two or more variables, emphasising highest and lowest categories (frequencies are normally displayed vertically and categories horizontally) compare the trends for two or more variables over time (frequencies are normally displayed vertically and discrete time periods horizontally)
Pictogram	emphasise highest and lowest categories for one variable
Stacked bar chart	compare frequency of occurrence for two or more variables, emphasising the variables' totals (frequencies are normally displayed vertically and categories horizontally)
Percentage component bar chart	compare proportions in each variable category for two or more variables (proportions are normally displayed vertically and categories horizontally)
Comparative pie chart	compare proportions in each variable category for two or more variables
Comparative proportional pie chart	compare proportions in each variable category and relative totals for two or more variables

Bar charts or graphs

Bar charts or graphs are especially useful when you want to emphasise the highest and lowest values of a variable. With a bar chart, each category within the variable is represented by a rectangular bar, and the frequency of occurrence is shown by the height (or length) of the bar. Each bar is separated from adjacent bars by a gap, emphasising that the categories are distinct. This means that, as well as categorical variables such as nationality, gender and religion, you can use a bar chart to represent discrete variables provided there are not too many categories! Figure 4.1 shows a bar chart created for the data in Table 4.1 using Excel's Chart Wizard.

Figure 4.1 Bar chart
The event was value for money

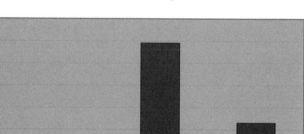

However, whilst you might feel that this graph is acceptable for a report or presentation, it would benefit from adding a more easily understandable label for each of the axes, a clearer title and stating the source of the data it contains. In addition, its visual presentation could be improved using the Excel software (see Figure 4.2). Remember our rule of thumb: your graph should be clear enough to allow it to be understood without having to read any of your text!

Figure 4.2   Annotated bar chart for a report

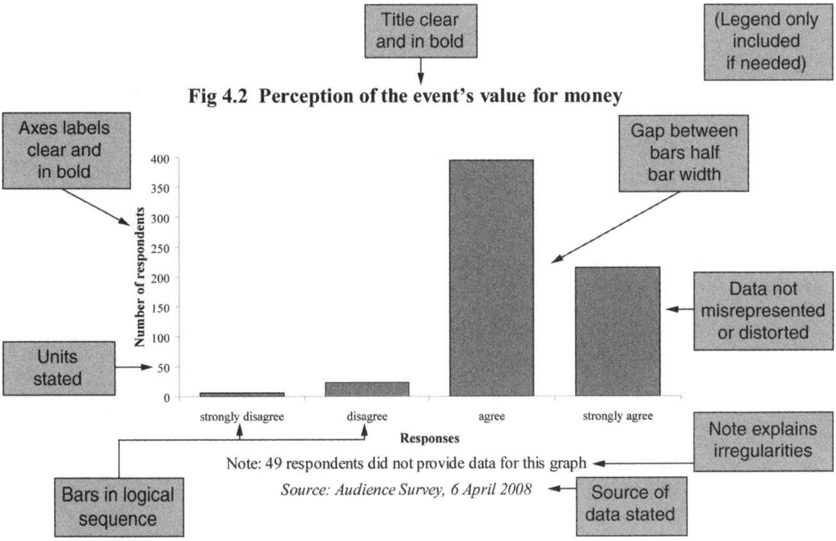

Bar charts can also be used when you want to compare the frequency of occurrence between two or more categorical data variables. This is done using a multiple bar chart (Figure 2.3), as already discussed in Chapter 2.

Pie charts

Pie charts are used when you wish to show the proportion of a variable in each category. The total for the data is represented by the area of the circle ('pie'), and each category's share of the total is represented by the area of a segment of that circle (i.e. a 'slice' of the 'pie'). The advantage of a pie chart is that it easy to compare the areas represented by the slices of the pie visually, but it is only useful if the number of categories is small, say no more than eight segments. When drawing a pie chart, it is helpful to shade those segments that are smaller in a darker colour.

Figure 4.3   Annotated pie chart for a report

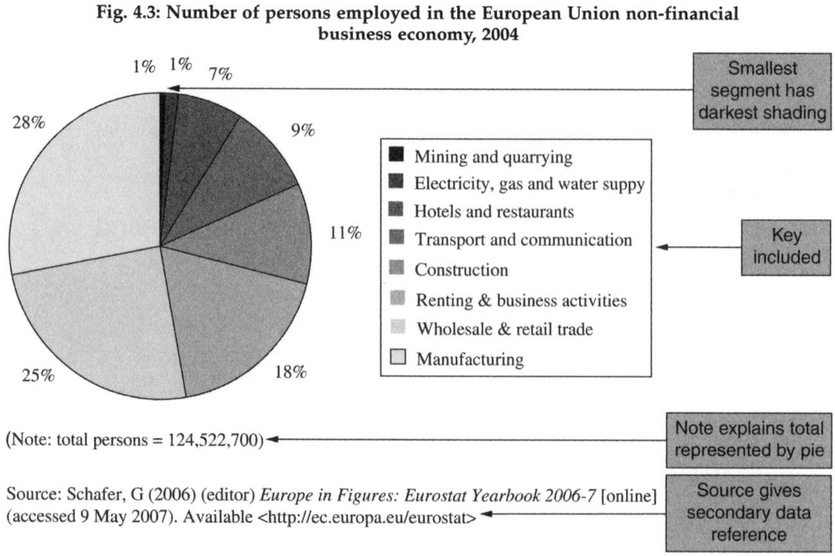

Fig. 4.3: Number of persons employed in the European Union non-financial business economy, 2004

Presenting numerical data using tables

Although it would be possible to present numerical data where the data values are discrete in a table, this is unlikely to be practicable – the large number of different values would make the table too large to interpret easily or indeed to fit on a page! To overcome this it is necessary to group the values for each variable into categories. This is always necessary for continuous data. Once you have grouped the data for your numerical variables they have, in effect, become categorical variables. This means you can present the data they contain as frequency tables and cross-tabulations, as discussed for categorical data.

Presenting numerical data using graphs

There are a wide range of graphs that are suitable for presenting numerical data. Those most frequently used are summarised in Table 4.5 along with when to use them. Those shaded in Table 4.5 are those graphs you are most likely to use. You will probably have less use for those graphs not shaded.

Table 4.5 Graphs for presenting numerical data and when to use them

Graph	Use when you want to present data to
Histogram	show frequency of occurrence and emphasise highest and lowest categories for one variable show the distribution of categories for one variable (frequencies are normally displayed vertically and categories horizontally and the data values will need to be grouped into categories)
Line graph	show the trend for one variable over time
Multiple line graph	compare the trends for two or more variables over time
Scatter graph	show the relationship between the individual cases for two variables
Frequency polygon	show frequency of occurrence and emphasise highest and lowest categories for one variable show the distribution of categories for one variable (frequencies are normally displayed vertically and categories horizontally, and the data values will need to be grouped into categories)
Box plot	show the distribution of values for one variable and present statistics such as the median, quartiles, range and inter-quartile range

Multiple box plot	compare the distribution of values for two or more variables and present statistics such as the median, quartiles, range and inter-quartile range

Histograms

Histograms are the numerical data equivalent of bar charts. They are especially useful when you want to emphasise the highest and lowest values or the distribution of values for a variable. Before drawing your histogram you will nearly always need to group your data into a series of groups along a continuous scale. This means you will need to:

(i)   decide on the classes into which to group the variable's data;

(ii)   create a frequency table recording the number of times values occur in each of these classes;

(iii)   draw your histogram using a bar to represent the frequency with which values occur in a class.

The main differences between the appearance of a bar chart and a histogram are as follows:

● The horizontal axis has a continuous scale, and is represented by the bars of data being joined together.

● The area, not the height, of each bar represents the frequency. This is extremely important if you are using classes of different sizes.

The frequency table in Table 4.6 records the length of talk time given by mobile phone batteries selected at random from a production line, charged and then used until they no longer worked. Within this table we chose to make all the classes the same size, 20 minutes. This made drawing the histogram (Figure 4.4) easier as the bars were all the same width and is something worth remembering, as most statistical software cannot draw histograms with unequal class sizes.

Table 4.6 Talk time from mobile phone batteries tested

Class	Frequency
40 to under 60 minutes	2
60 to under 80 minutes	9
80 to under 100 minutes	13
100 to under 120 minutes	14
120 to under 140 minutes	8
140 to under 160 minutes	4

Source: random testing, March 2008

Figure 4.4 Annotated histogram for a report

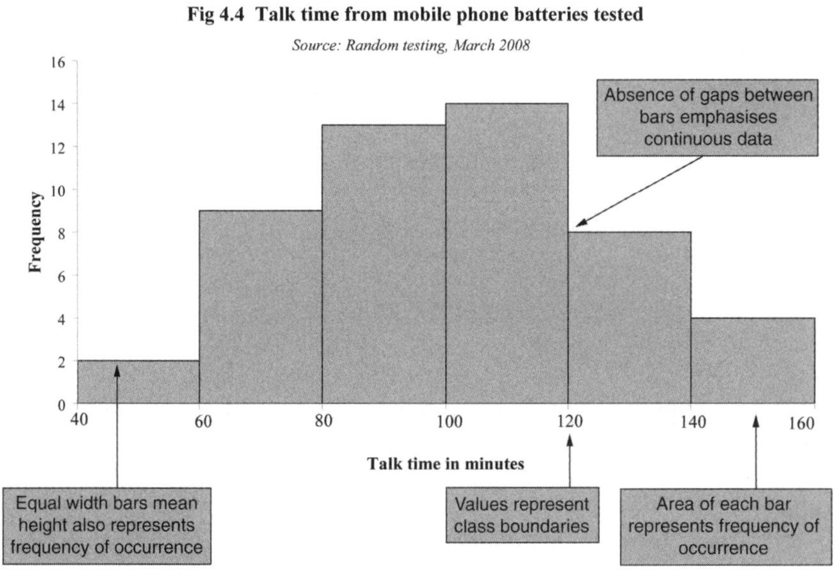
Fig 4.4 Talk time from mobile phone batteries tested
Source: Random testing, March 2008
16
14
12
10
8
6
4
2
0
Frequency
40
60
80
100
120
140
160
Talk time in minutes
Absence of gaps between bars emphasises continuous data
Equal width bars mean height also represents frequency of occurrence
Values represent class boundaries
Area of each bar represents frequency of occurrence

Line graphs and multiple line graphs

Line graphs should be used when you want to present what is happening over time, the trend being represented by the line. On line graphs, the horizontal axis is used to represent time, and the vertical axis the frequency, the data values for the time periods being joined by a line. Figure 4.5, created in Excel, shows the change in annual new registrations of motorcycles in the UK over the period 1995–2004, 2004 being the most recent year for which data were available when we were writing this book. When you want to compare trends for two or more variables over time, you just plot an additional line for each additional variable.

Figure 4.5   Annotated line graph for a report

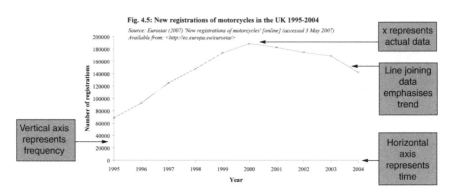

Source: Adapted from Eurostat (2007) New Registrations of Motorcycles. © *European Communities 2007. Reproduced with permission.*

Scatter graphs

Scatter graphs, also called scatter plots, are used to show the relationship between two numerical variables. Where you have an independent and a dependent variable, the horizontal axis is used to represent the independent variable (the one that is the variable manipulated (altered or changed) to find out its effect on another variable) and the vertical axis to represent the dependent variable (the one that is measured in response to the manipulation of the independent variable). However, you can use scatter plots to show relationships where you do not know which variable is dependent and which is independent. Each case's position on the graph is plotted against the two variables, normally being represented by a cross. The strength of any relationship is represented by the closeness of the crosses plotted to an imaginary straight line. Figure 4.6, created in Excel, shows the relationship between distance in miles (independent variable) and delivery time in minutes (dependent variable) for a home delivery pizza company.

Figure 4.6 Annotated scatter graph for a report

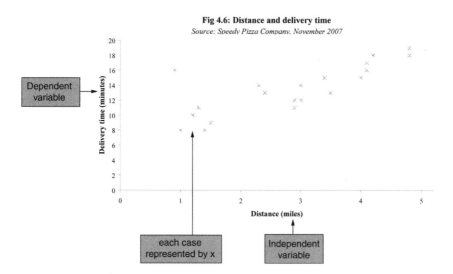

Final comments

You will no doubt have noticed that we have not included any three-dimensional graphs in this chapter. This is because we believe that they do not present data as clearly as two-dimensional graphs. If you are not sure what we mean, just compare Figure 4.7, with Figure 4.3 and ask yourself the question: which of the two pie charts represents the data for each sector without possible visual distortion?

Figure 4.7 Three-dimensional pie chart

Fig. 4.7: Number of persons employed in the European Union non-financial business economy, 2004

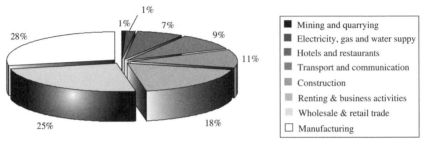

(Note: total persons = 124,522,700)

Source: Schäfer, G (ed.) (2007) *Europe in Figures: Eurostat Yearbook 2006-07* [online] (accessed 9 May 2007). Available from <http://ec.europa.eu/eurostat>

Source: adapted from Schäfer, G. (2007) Europe in Figures: Eurostat Yearbook 2006–07. © European Communities 2007. Reproduced with permission.

Chapter 5

Describing data

One of the first things you will need to do when analysing your data is to describe it statistically. This chapter outlines descriptive statistics you should use as well as how to use statistics to describe trends.

Because you are bound to have a great deal of data, you will need to summarise them. The way to do this is to use descriptive statistics. These statistics will tell you some straightforward, but often very useful things, and will enable you to describe and compare your variables numerically.

One of the first things that you will need to find out is the distribution of your data, that is, the overall relationship between a variable's values and their frequencies, called the **frequency distribution** (Chapter 4). While a bar chart will give clear information about the distribution of a single variable, you may need to be able to compare distributions of different variables that you have taken from different groups of respondents or from secondary data sets. Different variables can be compared by using summary or **descriptive statistics**. These give you two different pieces of information – the location and spread of your data. As a result, you can discover where the centre of your data is and how the data are spread around this centre. Thus, descriptive statistics will supply you with two types of information about your data – measures of location and measures of dispersion.

- **Measures of location** describe what is 'common', 'middling' or 'average' for a variable. The generic term for this is the **central tendency**; that is, the tendency of a frequency distribution to cluster around a single value or band of values. Depending upon the type of data, the most common ways to measure a variable's location are the mode, the median, and the arithmetic mean.

● **Measures of dispersion** or **spread** describe the spread or variability of data values for a numerical data variable. The dispersion of the data concerns how much the data values are spread out, what the limits of this spread are, whether the spread is even or not, and whether there are noticeable clusters. The more common measures of dispersion are the range, the inter-quartile range and the standard deviation, variance and kurtosis.

The two major types of data, categorical and numerical, use different measures of location and dispersion. Those you are likely to use are shaded in Tables 5.1 and 5.3, and we have structured this chapter to reflect this. In addition, we have included a section on describing trends over time along with an associated table of statistics (Table 5.7).

Describing the location of categorical data variables

Table 5.1 Statistics for describing categorical data and when to use them

Statistic	Use when you want to describe data by measuring the
mode	location (central tendency), stating the most frequently occurring category or categories for one variable
one-sample chi-square test	dispersion (spread), stating whether there is a statistically significant difference between the observed distribution pattern of data between categories for one variable and that which would have been expected if there was no pattern

You will have probably noticed that this section, like Table 5.1, is extremely short. This is because there is only one statistic that you need to know about when describing the location of categorical data, the mode.

Mode

The **mode** is the most frequently occurring category or categories for a data set. It is the category within a variable which occurs most often, and which therefore has the greatest frequency of occurrence. The mode is the simplest measure of location. When you want to identify, say, the most common or popular thing or event in your data, the mode will tell you – for instance, which colour is the most common in this year's sales of women's winter coats or a brand of car or type of chocolate bar, or which is the most popular of type of cultural attraction in a particular town, or which of the city's car parks is the most used. If you were looking at the frequency distribution of a variable using a bar chart, then the mode (or modal value) would be the tallest bar.

Data may have more than one mode, and this would enable you to find, say, the two most common colours of this year's winter coats or cars. In your bar chart, two separate bars with an equal maximum height would give you a **bimodal distribution**, and logically, if there were more than two bars with equal maximum height, then you would have a **multimodal distribution**.

When you have categorical data, because the only quantification possible is the number count of each category, you are restricted to the use of the mode as a measure of location. However, this does not mean you should use the mode only as a measure of location for categorical data. It is perfectly possible and often sensible to calculate the mode for numerical variables – for example, the modal number of children in a household is 2.

Describing the dispersion of categorical data variables

Like the section above describing the location of categorical data variables, this section is also is extremely short. Once again, there is only one statistic that you need to know about when describing the dispersion of categorical data, the one-sample chi-square test. This is probably one of the most widely used statistics for categorical data and is denoted by χ^2 (chi-square), where χ is the lower-case Greek letter 'chi' (pronounced 'ky'). We mention it here, but will explain it in more detail in Chapter 6. It is particularly useful in analysing categorical data, but can be used for data at other levels of measurement, for example by grouping numerical data into categories.

One-sample chi-square test

The **one-sample chi-square test** is used typically when you have data for a variable grouped into two or more categories (for example, Table 4.1). It is used when you want to discover whether there are statistically significant differences between the observed distribution pattern of data in your frequency distribution and that which we would have expected to see if there was no pattern. Consequently, you could use it to discover whether or not the hypothesis 'Dogs do express a significant preference for a brand of dog food' can be accepted. To test this hypothesis using the one-sample chi-square test, you would compare the observed distribution of preferences for brands of dog food with that which you would have expected to see if there was no preference (Table 5.2).

Table 5.2   Annotated frequency table of observed and expected data values

Data distribution observed		A	B	C		Data distribution that would have been expected if there was no preference
	1		Dogs' preferences			
	2		Observed	Expected		
	3	Brand A	140	125		
	4	Brand B	115	125		
	5	Brand C	145	125		
	6	Brand D	100	125		
	7	Total	500	500		

If the value of the chi-square test calculated using the table of data was significant then your null hypothesis that 'Dogs do not express a significant preference for a brand of dog food' could be rejected. In rejecting the null hypothesis you would be saying that the observed distribution of data in your frequency distribution differs significantly from that which you would have expected to see if there was no preference. We will discuss hypothesis testing and the chi-square test in more detail in Chapter 6. For the moment, it is important that you remember that the chi-square test only gives sensible results if the assumptions of the statistic are met, another aspect we talk about in Chapter 6.

Describing the location of numerical data variables

Table 5.3 Statistics for describing numerical data and when to use them

Statistic	Use when you want to describe data by measuring the
median	location (central tendency), stating the middle data value of the set of ranked data values for one variable
(arithmetic) mean	location (central tendency), stating the average data value of the set of data values for one variable
mode	location (central tendency), stating the most frequently occurring value or values for one variable
range	dispersion (spread), stating the difference between the highest and lowest ranked data values for one variable
inter-quartile range	dispersion (spread), stating the difference within the middle 50% of ranked data values for one variable
standard deviation	dispersion (spread), stating the extent to which the data values for one variable are spread around its mean using the same units as those in which the data were recorded
variance	dispersion (spread), stating the extent the data values for one variable are spread around its mean, but in the square of the units in which the data were recorded

| skewness | dispersion (spread), stating how the shape of the distribution of the data values for a variable deviates from a symmetrical (normal) distribution |
| kurtosis | dispersion (spread), stating how the pointedness or flatness of the shape of the distribution of the data values for a variable differs from the bell-like (normal) distribution |

As you can see from Table 5.3, statistics for describing numerical data are more numerous. The most frequently used measures of location (central tendency) are, in order, the mean and the median, although, as we have already seen, you can also use the mode as a measure of location for numerical data.

Median

The **median** is the middle value in a set of ranked data values, so that half the cases fall above and half the cases fall below it. When the distribution has an even number of values, the median is the average (mid-point) of the two middle values. If the total number of values is odd, then the median is the value in the middle (Table 5.4).

You would use the median when, for example, you wanted to find the typical salary in a firm – not the average (mean) salary, but the amount that is in the middle of your data set of salaries. Calculating the median for a variable is not complicated:

1. Put all the values in ascending rank order from smallest to largest.

2. If the number of values is odd, the one that is exactly in the middle is the median.

3. If the number of values is even, then:

    (a) take the two values that appear either side of the middle;

    (b) add them together;

    (c) divide by 2, and you have the median.

Table 5.4   Annotated table showing the median salary for a
group of employees

	A	B	C
1	**Name**	**Annual Salary £**	**Rank**
2	Fred	17408	1
3	Norman	17408	2
4	Mia	17408	3
5	Jason	18398	4
6	Tracey	18398	5
7	Elspeth	20850	6
8	Jamine	20850	7
9	Veronica	23790	8
10	Alice	29130	9
11	Grenville	35178	10
12	Dave	44603	11

Note: values are in rank order

Middle value

Median salary

The median isn't affected by **outliers** (the statistical term for values that are extremely high or extremely low compared with the rest of the data for a variable) in the way that the mean is. The median is generally a more useful measure of location than the mode for numeric data.

(Arithmetic) mean

The **mean** is probably the most commonly used statistic to find out where the 'centre' of your data is. It includes all data values in its calculation and is represented by the symbol $\bar{x}$ ('x-bar') when it is the mean of a sample and by μ, the lower-case Greek letter 'mu', when it is the mean of a population.

You calculate the mean whenever you need to know what is usually called the 'average' of the data values for a variable. The mean is the building block for the statistical tests that you will use in order to explore relationships, and it tends to be the value that the readers of your research will be looking for. However, you should only calculate the mean if you have variables measured at interval or ratio levels. This is one of the statistical rules that tends to get ignored, and our advice to you is that you should consult your supervisor should you wish to ignore the rule.

Calculating the mean is simple. All you need to do (or, if you prefer, get a calculator or statistical software to do for you) is:

1. Add up all the values in your data variable – say the salaries of your respondents.
2. Divide this total by the number of values in the variable.

What you need to look out for, however, is that in this instance, and in others like it, the mean can be somewhat misleading. It might be that one or two of the respondents (perhaps because they are the most senior executives) have salaries very much larger than most of the rest of the employees. Outliers of extremely high numbers will force the value of the mean upward, and extremely low numbers will force the value of the mean downward. Consequently, if you have outliers, the mean doesn't really represent the average of the respondents' salaries.

The mean of a data set will be affected by outliers, although the median is not. Whether you put both of these statistics into your report of your results or you choose to use only the most relevant one, you may well find it useful to calculate both the mean and the median. You can then compare the two statistics and this will give you a better feel for what is 'happening' in your data.

Comparing means with medians

This is where the reputation of statistics as 'shifty' or 'dodgy' comes in. We've said that you need to use statistics appropriately, and the trouble is that 'appropriately' is itself a somewhat slippery term.

When it comes to salaries, for instance, if you want to show how much the organisation is paying everyone, and you want to include those managers who are earning very much higher salaries than most of the other employees, then you will want to report the mean. But, if you were the interested in the perspective of the non-managerial employees, then you would be interested in the median, as this represents what the employees in the middle of the range of salaries are earning. Having calculated the median, you will then know that 50% of employees earn more than the median, and 50% earn less. Therefore, both the mean and the median are 'appropriate', but only according to your research purpose. You need to make absolutely clear where your interest lies, so that your examiner understands that you have used the right statistic for your purpose.

Describing the dispersion of numerical data variables

For numerical data variables it is not enough just to describe the central tendency using a statistic. You will also need to describe how the data values are dispersed from or cluster around the measure of location you have used. As can be seen from Table 5.3, this is commonly done using one or more of the following three statistics:

- the range, which is the difference in data values for a numerical variable between the lowest and the highest;
- the inter-quartile range, which is the difference in data values for a numerical variable within the middle 50% of values;
- the standard deviation, which describes the extent to which values for a numerical variable differ from the mean.

Range

The **range** describes the full extent of variability of the spread (dispersion) of data values, in an interval or ratio variable. It is the difference between the lowest and highest values so, although the range records the full variability in the data, it ignores all the data values other than these two. This means the remaining data values have no influence on the statistic at all.

Inter-quartile range

The **inter-quartile range**, also called the **mid spread**, describes the variability of the spread (dispersion) for the middle 50% of ranked data values for a numerical variable. The boundaries to the middle

50% of ranked data values are represented by the **lower quartile** (located a quarter (25%) of the way through the ranked data values starting at the lowest value) and the **upper quartile** (located three quarters (75%) of the way through the ranked data values starting at the lowest value). Half of your data values will fall between the upper and lower quartiles. The difference between the upper and lower quartiles is the inter-quartile range. In other words, it is concerned only with the middle 50% of the data values, and ignores extreme values (Table 5.5).

Table 5.5 Annotated table showing the inter-quartile range for the age of a group of employees

	A	B	C	
1	**Name**	**Age**	**Rank**	Note: values are in rank order
2	Mary	16	1	
3	Greg	19	2	
4	Steve	19	3	
5	Valentine	20	4	
6	Ashraf	22	5	Lower quartile is ¾ of way between 4th and 5th value
7	Sarah	23	6	
8	Mohammad	24	7	**Lower quartile** is ¾ of way between 20 and 22 = **21.5 years**
9	Hoza	24	8	
10	Peter	26	9	
11	Phil	27	10	
12	Liam	29	11	
13	Jane	29	12	
14	Marie	30	13	
15	Benji	33	14	Upper quartile is ¼ of way between 14th and 15th value
16	Jemma	38	15	
17	Kylie	40	16	
18	Fern	49	17	**Upper quartile** is ¼ of way between 33 and 38 = **34.25 years**
19	Josie	56	18	

Inter-quartile range = 34.25 − 21.5 = **12.75 years**

The inter-quartile range is used with numerical data in conjunction with the median. It is can also be used with numerical data if you suspect that you have a non-symmetrical (**asymmetrical**) distribution (more of which later in this chapter). Using the inter-quartile range overcomes the problem of the inclusion of extreme values, which happens when calculating the range, because this measures the spread of the data around the median, ignoring values beyond the lower and upper quartiles.

In working out the lower and upper quartiles, you are calculating the values that are precisely one quarter and three quarters of the way through your ranked data. These values often fall between two data values (Table 5.5). When this happens, you will need to calculate the precise lower or upper quartile rather than just record an existing data value. The calculated value will be either one quarter, half, or three quarters of the way between the two values that appear on either side. To calculate the precise position of the quartiles, proceed as follows:

1. Add 1 to the total number of values in your ranked data (for the data in Table 5.5, 18 + 1 = 19).
2. (a) For the lower quartile, multiply this number by ¼ (for Table 5.5, 19 × ¼ = 4¾).
    (b) For the upper quartile, multiply this number by ¾ (for Table 5.5, 19 × ¾ = 14¼).
3. The answers in 2 point to the precise position of the quartiles:
    (a) for Table 5.5, the lower quartile is ¾ of the way between the 4th and 5th values of 20 and 22, that is, 21½ years;
    (b) for Table 5.5, the upper quartile is ¼ of the way between the 14th and 15th values of 33 and 38, that is, 34¼ years.

Standard deviation

The **standard deviation** describes the extent of spread of data values for a variable around the mean. It is used when you want to describe how far away from a numerical variable's mean (average) the data values typically are. It is perhaps the most frequently used measure of dispersion, because it improves your ability to interpret the data by expressing deviations in their original units (e.g. profit in euros, distance in metres). It is also important as a descriptive statistic because it describes the amount of variability of the individual values within a data variable.

If you are going to describe a variable using the standard deviation, there are two standard deviations to choose from:

- the standard deviation of the entire population of data, denoted by the lower-case Greek letter σ 'sigma';

- the standard deviation of a sample from the population of data, which is denoted by the letter *s* (statistical software often labels this 'SD' or 'sd').

Mostly, when researchers use the term 'standard deviation', they mean the standard deviation of a sample because data are rarely collected for the entire population.

As in so much else where statistics are concerned, whether or not you want a small or a large standard deviation depends on what you are measuring. Parts for a machine, for instance, need to be accurate in order to fit, and so the less they vary the better, while it is probably of less concern to your research if the salaries of the firm you are interested in vary a great deal.

It is often helpful to look at the standard deviation together with the mean. This will enable you to describe how the data for a variable are dispersed around the mean for a **normal distribution**, that is, one where the data have a bell-shaped frequency curve (Figure 5.1). The **empirical rule** is useful here. It states that for approximately normally distributed data, around 68% of the data lie within one standard deviation (either side) of the mean, about 95% of the data lie within two standard deviations of the mean, and nearly all of the data lie within three standard deviations of the mean (Figure 5.1). You are unlikely to be concerned with virtually all of the data values in your variable, and will be happy to settle for 95%. It is probably not worthwhile to go two more standard deviations on either side of the mean to pick up the extra 5% of the data.

For example, to describe the delivery time data for the Speedy Pizza Company you would calculate the mean and the standard deviation (Table 5.6). Using these data, you could say that 68% of the

Figure 5.1 Applying the empirical rule to normally distributed data

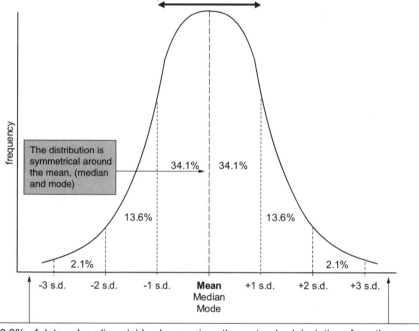

99.7% of data values lie within plus or minus three standard deviations from the mean

95.4% of data values lie within plus or minus two standard deviations from the mean

68.3% of data values lie within plus or minus one standard deviation from the mean

frequency

The distribution is symmetrical around the mean, (median and mode)

34.1%   34.1%

13.6%   13.6%

2.1%   2.1%

-3 s.d.   -2 s.d.   -1 s.d.   **Mean**   +1 s.d.   +2 s.d.   +3 s.d.
                                      Median
                                      Mode

0.3% of data values lie outside plus or minus three standard deviations from the mean

time pizzas would be delivered within approximately 10–17 minutes, and 95% of the time pizzas would be delivered within approximately 6–20 minutes.

Like the mean, the standard deviation is affected by outlying data values. If your data have outliers on the upper end, you will find that shape represented by a graph (Figure 5.1 is called a frequency polygon) in which the frequency of data values is skewed to the right, and the mean will usually be larger than the median. If the data have outliers on the lower end, the frequency of the data values will be skewed to the left, and the mean will usually be smaller than the

Table 5.6 Annotated table showing the mean
and standard deviation

	A	B	C	D	E	
1	Distance (miles)	Delivery time (minutes)				
2	3.5	13				
3	2.4	13				
4	4.8	19				
5	4.2	18				
6	3	12				
7	1.3	11		Delivery time		68% of pizzas are
8	1	8		Mean =	13.45	delivered within the
9	3	14				mean (13.45 minutes)...
10	1.5	9				
11	4.1	16		Delivery time		...plus or minus one
12	3.4	15		S.d. =	3.332061	standard deviation
13	2.3	14				(3.33 minutes)
14	4.8	18				
15	4.1	17				In other words, 68%
16	2.9	11				of pizzas are delivered
17	1.2	10				between 10.12 minutes
18	0.9	16				and 16.78 minutes;
19	2.9	12				say between 10 and
20	1.4	8				17 minutes.
21	4	15				

median. And if the data are symmetric as in Figure 5.1 (have the same shape on either side of the middle), then the mean and the median will be the same.

Variance

The variance is also a measure of how much the data values for a numerical variable differ from (are dispersed about) the mean. However, although statistics textbooks will often say that you should use the variance with numerical data, it is rarely used in research reports as a statistic in its own right. This is because the statistic's value is expressed in terms of the square of the data values and not the data values themselves. This makes any interpretation very difficult as, rather that talking about say, profit in euros, the variance would relate to euros^2. You should use the standard deviation, which is the square root of the variance. This means your profit is no longer in euros^2, but is in euros.

Skewness and kurtosis

We mention these here, so that you will have the complete picture. These two statistics can be used to describe the shape of the distribution of a variable's data values. However, we suspect that you can manage without them.

Skewness is a measure of how the shape of the distribution of a variable's data values deviates from a symmetrical (normal) distribution. In a symmetrical distribution (Figure 5.1), the mean, median and mode are in the same location. A distribution that has cases stretching out towards one side or the other (this is called a **tail**) is said to be skewed. When a tail stretches to the left, to the smaller values, it is termed a **negatively skewed** distribution. Often when this happens, the value of the mean is smaller than that of the median, which is smaller than that of the mode. A tail stretching toward the right, to the larger values, is termed a **positively skewed** distribution; often with the mean being larger than the median which is larger than the mode (Figure 5.2).

Kurtosis measures the pointedness or flatness of the shape of the distribution of a variable's data values relative to the bell-like shape of a normal distribution. However, from a practical standpoint, other than providing graphs like those in Figure 5.2 to demonstrate the shape of your data, should you wish to do so, you are unlikely to need to calculate either the skewness or the kurtosis statistics for a data variable.

Figure 5.2 Annotated graphs illustrating skewness and kurtosis

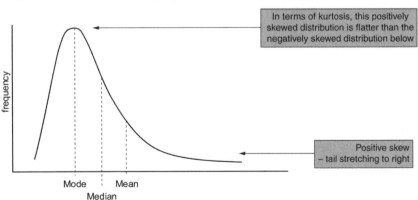

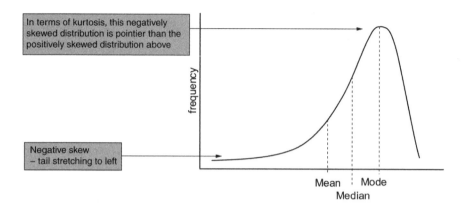

In terms of kurtosis, this negatively skewed distribution is pointier than the positively skewed distribution above

Negative skew – tail stretching to left

Mean Mode
Median

Describing trends for numerical data variables

We have already seen in Chapter 4 how a line graph can be used to show a trend. If you have numerical data that have been collected over time and wish to describe statistically the trend for a variable relative to a particular period such as a year, you can do this by calculating a **simple index number** (Table 5.7). Index numbers are widely used in business publications and by businesses. The Financial Times share indices such as the FT-SE 100 and the All-Share Index track share prices, building societies such as the Nationwide regularly publish house price indices, and the Retail Price Index is used to show how much prices have changed. Index numbers allow relative changes to be explored and compared.

Table 5.7 Statistics for describing trends in numerical data and when to use them

Statistic	Use when you want to describe
Simple index number	the **relative change** in a series of values for a numerical variable over time (by calculating index numbers, comparisons can be made between variables of different magnitudes)
Average index	the average **relative change** in a series of values for a number of numerical variables over time

Weighted average index	the average **relative change** in a series of values for a number of numerical variables over time, individual variables within the index being weighted according to their relative importance
Time series analysis	the long-term or secular **trend** of a series of values for a numerical variable over time

The period with which the comparison is being made is called the **base period** and is nearly always represented by the value of 100. (A notable exception is the FT-SE 100 index, whose base is 1000.) Change relative to this base period is represented by values for other periods. If a value is below 100, this represents a decrease relative to the base period, whereas if the value is above 100 it represents a relative increase. Interpretation of simple index numbers such as those in Table 5.8 is relatively straightforward. However, you must remember that the index number is always comparing back to the base period, in this case 2002. In addition, the actual magnitude of different values is lost in the calculation of the index. You could also plot the index numbers on a multiple line graph (see Chapter 4) to aid interpretation.

Table 5.8 Prices and simple index numbers for two products
2002–2007

Product	Price/Index	2002	2003	2004	2005	2006	2007
A	Price (€)	21.00	23.00	24.50	26.00	27.00	27.50
	Index	100	116.67	119.52	123.81	128.57	130.95
B	Price (€)	410.00	550.00	690.00	700.00	700.00	690.00
	Index	100	134.15	168.29	170.73	170.73	168.29

Final comments

In order to create your questionnaire or interview schedule, you will have read research papers (or books) published on or around your topic. You will have found that authors undertook statistical analysis on their data, and in some instances you will notice that they have ignored the rules about which tests should be used on which types of data, and that perhaps they will have calculated means and standard deviations for ordinal or even nominal data rather than reserving them for interval and ratio data. This does not mean that you should do the same! Many researchers (perhaps including your supervisor) will object to your using such tests on your categorical data variables. It might therefore be helpful, if you discuss this issue with your supervisor when you have decided on the tests you wish to use.

Chapter 6

Inferring differences and relationships from data

This chapter explains, and provides advice about, statistical tests for inferring differences and relationships between variables.

Before looking at statistics to test for differences between and relationships between variables, we feel it is important to remind you that, before using any of these statistics, you will need to get to know your data by drawing tables and graphs (Chapter 4) and describing your data (Chapter 5).

We assume that you are undertaking statistical analysis because you wish to infer something about a population from the sample of data you have collected. Indeed if you have conducted a census of the entire population then statistical inference is unnecessary because any differences or relationships you find are true and do really exist. However, researchers rarely obtain data from the entire population and so you will almost certainly be forced to draw inferences from a sample using statistical tests.

Before we begin to discuss the tests you might choose to elicit these, we think it would be helpful to start this chapter by explaining two concepts associated with inferential statistics, probability and hypothesis testing (and you will find short definitions of these in the Glossary). Subsequently we will outline, with varying degrees of detail, the tests associated with inferring differences and relationships between categorical data variables and between numerical data variables. As we've said before, this book concentrates on the three Ws – which statistical test the use, when to use it, and why. We ignore the details of how to calculate them and how to use statistical analysis software, leaving these aspects for the statistics books that explain statistical techniques.

Probability and confidence

Within inferential statistics, reasoning moves from specific facts about your sample to inferring more general, but tentative, conclusions about the population from which your sample was selected. Probability estimates state the **likelihood** of what you have inferred about the population from your sample being true. Inferential statistics, therefore, are a way to apply inductive reasoning with some level of confidence, because they allow you to reason from evidence found in your sample to the conclusions you wish to make about the population.

Probability

Statistical probability uses everyday language in a special way. In statistics, **probability** is a number that represents the likelihood that a particular finding or relationship between variables (an event) will have occurred.

Informally, you will talk about probabilities as the percentage chance of something occurring or you use odds, such as a 3 to 1 chance of a horse winning a race. However, in statistics probabilities are expressed formally as decimal numbers between 0 and 1. A probability of 0 specifies that an event will never happen, whilst a probability of 1 specifies that an event will always happen. Statisticians express probabilities as inequalities, which means that the probability (represented by the lower-case letter p) of an event occurring (by chance) is written as:

$p <$ probability is less than ...
$p >$ probability is greater than ...
$p =$ probability is equal to ...
$p \leq$ probability is less than or equal to ...
$p \geq$ probability is greater than or equal to ...

a particular value. So a probability of less than 0.05 (5%) of an event occurring (by chance) would be expressed as $p < 0.05$.

As you might expect, there are rules governing the calculation of the probabilities of events, but this isn't the place to go into these details. The point is that you use probability to say how likely your findings are to have occurred by chance and, by doing this, indicate how much those reading your project can trust them.

Confidence

In statistics, the concept of 'confidence' has two aspects, the confidence level and the confidence interval. These allow you to say just how sure (**confidence level**) you are about your prediction or estimate of the population from your sample and how accurate (**confidence interval**) you believe your prediction to be.

For example, you may have collected data from a sample of consumers about their purchasing preferences and found that, if they were to go shopping today, 48% of them would purchase a particular product. Based on this you could say that 48% of consumers (the total population) will purchase the product. In your project report you could qualify this prediction by saying that you were 95% certain (your confidence level) that the prediction was accurate to within plus or minus 2% (your confidence interval). The term '95% certain' means that you are confident that the value calculated from your sample data plus or minus the confidence interval will represent that of the true population 95% of the times it is used. The confidence interval, in this example 'plus or minus 2%', gives an accuracy to the value you have calculated from these data. Consequently, for this example, your confidence interval is 48% plus or minus 2%, in other words between 46% and 50%.

Remember that you have no guarantee that the sample you select will give an accurate prediction or estimation. By using a 95% confidence level you are stating that you are confident that, if you selected 100 different samples from your population, then for 95 of these 100 samples your prediction or estimate of the population would be within the confidence intervals you state.

Hypotheses and statistical significance

Hypotheses

A **hypothesis** is a statement of, or a speculation about, the relationships among the variables that you intend to study. Statistically, hypotheses are testable statements or predictions about relationships or differences between variables, which, if statistically significant, will support a theory. For example, you may hypothesise that employees are more trusting of their organisation if they consider their line manager cares about them personally. If your organisational question-naire collects data from a sample of employees about how trusting they are of their organisation and the extent to which they consider their line manager cares about them personally, you can test this hypothesis statistically. By doing this you will establish the probabil-ity of such a relationship occurring by chance and, therefore, whether or not any relationship between these variables is statistically signifi-cant.

You are using inductive reasoning when you move from specific facts about your sample to general (but tentative) conclusions from those facts. Because you can never be completely sure about your inferences, you use probability estimates in order to qualify your results and state the likelihood of having reached the wrong conclu-sions. By using statistical inference, you are using the evidence you have found in your sample to come to a conclusion about the population. It is inferential statistics that enables the testing of statistical hypotheses.

The purpose of **hypothesis testing** is to find out the validity or otherwise of a hypothesis when you have collected data from a sample, rather than from the entire population. Since any sample will almost certainly vary somewhat from its population, we need to judge whether differences or relationships are statistically significant or only represent random fluctuations. Consequently, the significance of the hypothesis is evaluated by finding out the probability that the data you have collected reveal true patterns in the population from which they were drawn, rather than these patterns having occurred by chance alone.

It is also important for you to understand the counter-intuitive fact that statistical significance and practical significance are not synony-mous, and that while a small difference might have statistical signifi-cance, it might have no practical significance whatever. This is more likely to occur with large sample sizes, where even minor differences may be statistically significant.

Statistical significance

Testing for **statistical significance** is testing the probability of a relationship between two or more variables, defined by a hypothesis, occurring by chance alone. It is based on the premise that there is no difference between the sample and the population from which it was drawn. This means it is essential that your sample is representative of the population from which it is drawn.

Significance tests work on the premise of rejecting a hypothesis that there is no significant difference between, or no significant relationship between, two or more variables. This is known as the **null hypothesis** and represented by the upper-case letter H and the number zero (H_0). You reject the null hypothesis because, whilst it is impossible to prove definitively that there will always be a difference, it is possible to prove definitively that there will not always be no difference.

By rejecting a hypothesis of no difference or no relationship you are substantiating the opposite, and showing that there may be a significant difference or significant relationship. This can be likened to presuming that someone in a legal trial is innocent until they are proven guilty, that is, you have to statistically reject the assumption that the person is innocent. The statement that there is a significant difference or relationship, phrased as a hypothesis, is also known as the **alternative hypothesis**. This is symbolised by the upper case letter H and either the number one or the lower-case letter a (H_1 or H_a).

For instance, a null hypothesis (H_0) could be that there has been no change in the number of employees who have been absent from work over the past six months. The alternative hypothesis (H_1) could then be either that the number of employees absent has changed, or that the number of employees absent has increased (or decreased). You then calculate an appropriate test statistic and work out the probability of that statistic occurring by chance alone, which you can think of as the probability that the null hypothesis is likely to be true. While some software packages automatically calculate this probability precisely for you, others do not. If the software does not calculate the precise probability of the statistic occurring by chance alone, you will need to obtain what is termed the **critical value** for the test statistic. Critical values are recorded in tables for specified statistics and provide the criterion that defines whether or not your null hypothesis should be rejected. Tables of critical values for different test statistics can usually be found in statistics textbooks as appendices and allow you to ascertain the approximate probability of the statistic occurring by chance alone. If the critical value is larger, you cannot reject the null hypothesis. Usually, if the probability is higher than 0.05 ($p > 0.05$), then you do not reject the null hypothesis. This is because the likelihood of the null hypothesis being true is greater than 1 in 20. Sometimes statisticians choose not to reject the null hypothesis if the probability of it being true is greater than 1 in 100 ($p > 0.01$).

We have some interesting terminology here. In hypothesis testing the analysis may show that you cannot reject the null hypothesis. Notice that we do not say 'accept' but say 'not reject' the null hypothesis. This is where inductive reasoning comes in. Testing for statistical significance gives you only a chance either to reject (disprove) or to fail to reject the hypothesis. Not surprisingly, you will often hear people say or read in an article the phrase 'accept the null hypothesis'. This is because the correct version is clumsy – 'fail to reject the null hypothesis'.

If you reject a null hypothesis (finding a statistically significant difference), then you are accepting the alternative hypothesis. Of course, in either not rejecting or rejecting a null hypothesis, you can make incorrect decisions. You can accept (fail to reject) a null hypothesis when it should have been rejected, or reject it when it should have been accepted. Statisticians have specific terms for these mistakes. Rejecting a null hypothesis, when it is in reality correct and should not have been rejected, is called a **Type I error**. A Type I error can therefore be likened to a jury finding a person guilty when in reality they are innocent! Failing to reject a null hypothesis which is, in reality, incorrect is called a **Type II error**. This can be likened to a jury finding a person innocent when, in reality, they are guilty. Whilst both are miscarriages of justice, we would argue that the latter is preferable.

Testing

Testing for statistical significance follows a well-defined process, although you will find other authors offer a different number and sequence of steps.

1. *State your null hypothesis.* While you are likely to be interested in testing a hypothesis of some relationship or difference, you need to use the null hypothesis of no relationship or difference for statistical testing purposes. This states what you believe, until evidence proves otherwise.

2. *Choose a statistical test.* It hardly needs to be said that to test a hypothesis, you must choose an appropriate statistical test for your type of data and for what you wish to test. We will talk about these later in this chapter.

3. *Select the critical level of significance.* The most common critical level is 0.05, although sometimes 0.01 is used as the probability below which the null hypothesis will no longer be accepted as being true.

4. *Calculate the test statistic.* Use your statistical software to calculate an appropriate test statistic.

5. *Interpret the calculated probability value or the critical test value.* After you have obtained the test statistic, depending upon the software package you have used, you may need to obtain and interpret the critical value in the appropriate table for that statistic. Alternatively, the software package may report the probability (p value) of a sample as extreme as, or more extreme than, the value actually observed, given that the null hypothesis is true. The probability can then be compared with the level of significance selected.

6. *Interpret the test statistic.* Having rejected or accepted the null hypothesis, you need to draw conclusions as to what this means. Remember, when you reject a null hypothesis, you talk about an alternative hypothesis being 'supported', rather than being 'proved'.

The two major types of data, categorical and numerical, use different statistics to infer differences and relationships between variables. Tests of significance for categorical data are termed **non-parametric tests**, whereas those used for numerical data are termed **parametric tests**. Statisticians generally talk about parametric tests as being more powerful because the data used in the calculation are interval or ratio. Those tests you are likely to use are shaded in Tables

6.1 and 6.4; the rest of this chapter is structured to reflect the distinction between categorical and numerical data and, consequently, non-parametric and parametric tests.

Inferring differences and relationships between categorical data variables

Non-parametric tests are used to test hypotheses with nominal data and are, technically, also the only correct tests to use with ordinal data. They are sometimes used with numerical data that have been grouped, although this wastes some of the detail available in the data. As can be seen from Table 6.1, non-parametric tests are used when you wish to infer association between two variables. These tests are not as complicated as they might seem, those that you are most likely to use falling into two groups of similar tests:

- chi-square test and Fisher's exact test;

- Spearman's rank correlation coefficient and Kendall's rank correlation coefficient.

These are shaded in Table 6.1.

Table 6.1 Statistics for inferring differences and relationships between categorical data variables and when to use them

Statistic	Use when you want to infer association between two
Chi-square test	categorical variables, by stating whether there is a statistically significant **difference** between the observed distribution pattern of data in a two-way table (in which the categories of one of the variables form the rows and the categories of the other variable form the columns) and that which would have been expected by chance

Fisher's exact test	nominal variables, by stating whether there is a statistically significant **difference** between the observed distribution pattern of data in a two-way table (in which the categories of one of the variables form two rows and the categories of the other variable form two columns) and that which would have been expected by chance
Mann–Whitney *U*-test	ordinal variables, by stating whether the **difference** between the location of the two groups is statistically significant; that is, significantly different from that which would have been expected by chance
Kolmogorov–Smirnov test	ordinal variables, by stating whether the **differences** in the location and shape of the distribution of the two groups are statistically significant; that is, significantly different from that which would have been expected by chance
Spearman's rank correlation coefficient	ordinal variables, by assessing the strength of a **relationship** through the level of agreement between the two sets of rankings (being more appropriate if a variable does not contain tied ranks) and its statistical significance; that is, the likelihood of it having occurred by chance
Kendall's rank correlation coefficient	ordinal variables, by assessing the strength of a **relationship** through the level of agreement between the two sets of rankings (being more appropriate if a variable contains tied ranks) and its statistical significance; that is, the likelihood of it having occurred by chance

Chi-square test and Fisher's exact test

The chi-square test is, as we discovered in Chapter 5, probably the most widely used non-parametric test of (statistical) significance. When used to infer association between two categorical variables, it is occasionally referred to as the **two-sample chi-square test**. The latter name distinguishes it from the one-sample chi-square test we talked about in Chapter 5. It is particularly useful for nominal data collected from a sample, but can be used for data collected using higher levels of measurement if these data are grouped into categories.

The **chi-square test** calculates whether the difference between the observed distribution pattern of data collected from a sample shown in a two-way table (in which the categories of one of the variables form the rows and the categories of the other variable form the columns) is significantly different from that which would have been expected, based upon the null hypothesis. In other words, you compare the tabulated values for your sample with those you would have expected if there had been no underlying relationship between the two variables and then calculate the probability of a sample as extreme as, or more extreme than, that actually observed to have occurred. If this is less than 0.05 ($p < 0.05$) then the null hypothesis is usually rejected and you can say that the hypothesis that there is a significant difference is supported.

The chi-square statistic must be calculated using the observed values in the table, rather than percentages, and for the statistic to be reliable the following must also be true (statisticians refer to any such statement about data which needs to be true if the statistic is to be reliable as an **assumption**):

- the categories in the two-way table are mutually exclusive;
- no more than 20% of the cells in the two-way table can have expected values of less than 5.

Fortunately, statistical software packages such as SPSS, as well as calculating the value of the chi-square statistic and its significance, also automatically calculate the proportion of expected values that are less than 5 (Table 6.2). If this is greater than 20%, as in Table 6.2, the usual solution is to combine rows and/or columns, as long as this produces meaningful data. Unless this is done, the chi-square statistic cannot be used to decide whether to reject the null hypothesis as the test's assumptions have not been satisfied. Consequently, in Table 6.2 you would be unable to use the chi-square statistic to decide whether or not to reject the null hypothesis as 25% of the cells in your table have an expected value of less than 5.

Table 6.2 Annotated frequency table and chi-square test

			Gender * Is easy to book tickets Crosstabulation					
Table of data on which chi-square test is calculated				Is easy to book tickets				
				Strongly Disagree	Disagree	Agree	Strongly Agree	Total
Count = observed value	Gender	Female	Count	6	8	259	183	456
			Expected Count	6.2	9.0	246.4	194.3	456.0
Expected Count = expected value		Male	Count	3	5	96	97	201
			Expected Count	2.8	4.0	108.6	85.7	201.0
	Total		Count	9	13	355	280	657
			Expected Count	9.0	13.0	355.0	280.0	657.0

	Chi-Square Tests			
Chi-square statistic		Value	df	Asymp. Sig. (2-sided)
	Pearson Chi-Square	4.681[a]	3	.197
	Likelihood Ratio	4.666	3	.198
Proportion of cells having expected values of less than 5	Linear-by-Linear Association	1.933	1	.164
	N of Valid Cases	657		

Probability of the observed values in table occurring by chance (significance)

a. 2 cells (25.0%) have expected count less than 5. The minimum expected count is 2.75.

   Fisher's exact test is used instead of a chi-square test when you have nominal data in a table of two rows and two columns and if the expected values are too small to satisfy the assumptions of the chi-square test. Like the chi-square test, **Fisher's exact test** calculates whether there is a statistically significant difference between the observed distribution pattern of data in a two-way table and that which would have been expected based upon the null hypothesis.

Spearman's and Kendall's rank correlation coefficients

When analysing data, you often need to establish the strength of relationship between two variables and the probability that the relationship has occurred by chance. When a change in one variable is accompanied by a change in another variable, we say that there is a correlation between the variables. As we said in Chapter 4, this does not mean that one variable causes a change in the other, only that they are related. For relationships where you know that a change in one variable is accompanied by a change in another variable and where you have ordinal data, you can use statistics such as Spearman's rank correlation coefficient and Kendall's rank correlation coefficient.

Both Spearman's rank correlation coefficient (represented by the lower-case letters r_s or ρ, the lower-case Greek letter 'rho') and Kendall's rank correlation coefficient (represented by τ, the lower-case Greek letter 'tau') measure the association between the rankings for two variables. These ranks may be based upon status, importance or some other factor such as aptitude or test results. The calculated **correlation coefficient** for both statistics provides us with a measure of the strength of the relationship between these two variables, taking a value somewhere between –1 and +1. For example, a correlation coefficient of:

–1   means a perfect negative correlative between the two variables (as the ranks for one variable increase, the ranks of the other decrease);

–0.8 means a strong negative correlation between the two variables (as the ranks for one variable increase, the ranks of the other decrease, although there is limited variability in this relationship);

–0.5 means a medium negative correlation between the two variables (as the ranks for one variable increase, the ranks of the other decrease, although there is some variability in this relationship);

–0.3 means a weak negative correlation between the two variables (as the ranks for one variable increase, the ranks of the other decrease, although there is considerable variability in this relationship);

0   means no correlation between the two variables;

0.3   means a weak positive correlation between the two variables (as the ranks for one variable increase, the ranks of the other increase, although there is considerable variability in this relationship);

0.5   means a medium positive correlation between the two variables (as the ranks for one variable increase, the ranks of the other increase, although there is some variability in this relationship);

0.8   means a strong positive correlation between the two variables (as the ranks for one variable increase, the ranks of the other increase, although there is limited variability in this relationship);

1   means a perfect positive correlative between the two variables (as the ranks for one variable increase, the ranks of the other increase).

Spearman's rank correlation coefficient is most frequently used to assess the strength of a relationship between the two sets of rankings (ordinal data). If you have two variables, one of which is ordinal and the other numerical, you will need to rank the numerical data before calculating the correlation coefficient. When doing this, be sure to rank the data the same way, for example ensuring that for both variables a ranking of 1 has the same meaning (Table 6.3) and that your data contain no or few tied ranks.

Table 6.3   Annotated spreadsheet table with ranked data

	A	B	C	D		
		Aptitude test result (%)	Aptitude (ranked)	Sales performance (ranked)	Aptitude test result as a percentage	
1	Employee					
2	Jane	95	1	4	Aptitude test result ranked, highest score = 1	
3	Emily	90	2	1		
4	Ceri	71	3	2		
5	Zack	70	4	3	Sales performance ranked, best performance = 1	
6	Brandon	67	5	6		
7	Jemma	64	6	5		
8	Ben	58	7.5	9	Two employees tied as 7th, rank =7.5 (halfway between 7th and 8th)	
9	Lily	58	7.5	8		
10	Rachel	50	9	7		
11	Robert	48	10	10		

As noted in Table 6.1, if your data contain tied ranks, you should use **Kendall's rank correlation coefficient** to assess the strength of a relationship between the two sets of rankings (ordinal data). The resulting correlation coefficient is interpreted in exactly the same way.

If your data are collected for a sample rather than a population, you will also need to calculate the probability of your correlation having occurred by chance, whichever of these two statistics you use. In other words, you will need to calculate the probability of a sample showing a relationship as extreme as, or more extreme than that you actually observed having occurred by chance. If this probability is less than 0.05 ($p < 0.05$) then the null hypothesis of no relationship is usually rejected and you can say that the hypothesis that the relationship, represented by the correlation coefficient, is supported. Fortunately, most statistical software calculates this probability at the same time as calculating the correlation coefficient.

Inferring differences and relationships between numerical data variables

Parametric tests are used to test hypotheses with numerical data. As can be seen from Table 6.4, parametric tests are used to infer association in two distinct ways:

- by stating the likelihood (probability) of any differences occurring by chance;
- by assessing the strength of a relationship (and the likelihood of this occurring by chance).

Those statistics that you are most likely to use are shaded in Table 6.4. These are not the only tests you could use, but are the most commonly used. You can easily find how to calculate them in a statistics textbook. However, before you use them, you need to make sure that your data satisfy the following assumptions:

1. The cases must be independent of each other. This means that the selection of any one case for your sample should not affect the chances of any other case being included in the sample.
2. The cases need to be drawn from normally distributed populations. This is not particularly important provided the sample size is more than 30.
3. The measurement scales must be at least interval, so that arithmetic operations can be used on the data, although even this assumption is sometimes ignored!

In addition, some tests also make assumptions about the variance. We will talk about this assumption in relation to the specific tests when it is necessary!

Table 6.4 Statistics for inferring differences, relationships and trends for numerical data variables and when to use them

Statistic	Use when you want to infer association between
Independent groups t-test	two distinct groups, by stating the likelihood of any differences between the values for a numerical variable for each of the two groups (defined by a separate variable) having occurred by chance alone
Paired t-test	two distinct groups, where the numerical data values are in pairs, one from each group, by stating the likelihood of any **difference** between the paired values from the two groups (each group's values being contained in a separate variable) having occurred by chance alone
Analysis of variance (ANOVA)	three or more distinct groups, by stating the likelihood of any **difference** between the values for a numerical variable for each of the groups (defined by a separate variable) having occurred by chance alone
Pearson's product moment correlation coefficient (PMCC)	a dependent and an independent numerical variable, by assessing the strength of a **relationship** through the level of agreement between the two sets of values and its statistical significance; that is, the likelihood of this having occurred by chance alone

(continued)

Coefficient of determination (regression coefficient)	a dependent and an independent numerical variable, by assessing the strength of a **cause-and-effect relationship** through the level of agreement between the two sets of values and its statistical significance; that is, the likelihood of this having occurred by chance alone
Coefficient of multiple determination (multiple regression coefficient)	a dependent numerical variable and two or more independent numerical variables, by assessing the strength of a **cause-and-effect relationship** through the level of agreement between the values of the dependent and independent variables and its statistical significance; that is, the likelihood of this having occurred by chance alone
Regression equation (regression analysis)	a dependent numerical variable's values by **prediction** from the values of one or more independent numerical variables and its statistical significance; that is, the likelihood of this having occurred by chance alone
Regression equation (regression analysis)	the long-term or secular **trend** of a series of data values for a dependent numerical variable over time and its statistical significance; that is, the likelihood of this having occurred by chance alone

Independent groups and paired *t*-tests

To infer the likelihood of two distinct groups being different, *t*-tests are used. They can be used when you wish to find out whether two independent groups differ significantly from each other in the values recorded for a numerical variable. They can also be used when you wish to see whether the values recorded for the individual cases in your sample differ before and after some form of intervention. This is done by comparing the difference between the means of the two groups and calculating the likelihood of the difference occurring by chance. The difference between the means of the two groups is represented by the t value, and the likelihood of it occurring by chance by the probability (p).

In addition to the assumptions already outlined, t-tests require the data in the two groups to have the same variance. This means that the data should have the same standard deviation. Fortunately, provided the two groups are of a similar size, many statisticians say that this assumption can be ignored! As we hinted earlier, the two groups which you are comparing will be defined in one of two ways. Each of these requires a different type of t-test:

- Data for a numerical variable that is divided into two independent groups, using a categorical variable (Table 6.5), require an independent groups t-test:
- Paired data that are recorded for two groups as two separate numerical variables (Table 6.6), require a paired t-test.

The likelihood of numerical data, such as salary (Table 6.5), for two independent groups being significantly different is calculated using an **independent groups t-test**. This compares the differences between the means for each of the two groups and calculates the probability that this difference occurred by chance. If this is low, it will be represented by a large t value and a probability of less than 0.05 ($p < 0.05$) and means there is a statistically significant difference.

Table 6.5   Annotated spreadsheet table with data for an independent groups t-test

	A	B	
Numerical variable records data for both groups	salary	gender	Categorical variable divides data into two groups
2	€ 36,912.00	1	
3	€ 38,019.00	1	
4	€ 48,162.00	1	
5	€ 46,758.00	1	
Salary of individuals is recorded in euros — 6	€ 44,074.00	2	
7	€ 41,544.00	2	Variable 'gender' is coded:
8	€ 40,335.00	1	1 = male
9	€ 38,019.00	1	2 = female
10	€ 36,912.00	2	

The likelihood of paired numerical data for two variables that measure the same thing but under different conditions, such as individuals' test scores before and after an intervention (Table 6.6), being significantly different is calculated using a **paired *t*-test**. This compares the differences between the means for each of the two variables and calculates the probability that this difference occurred by chance. If this is low, it will be represented by a large *t* value and a probability of less than 0.05 ($p < 0.05$) and means there is a statistically significant difference.

Table 6.6   Annotated spreadsheet table with data for a paired
t-test

	A	B	C	
	name	score before intervention	score after intervention	
1				
2	Jemma	76	81	
3	Jane	45	39	
4	Ben	34	47	
5	Mark	21	34	
6	Kenneth	56	76	
7	Elizabeth	87	92	
8	Pam	46	54	
9	Muriel	59	62	

Numerical variable records scores before intervention

Numerical variable records scores after intervention

Each row represents one case

Each pair of data relates to one case

Analysis of variance

Analysis of variance, often abbreviated to ANOVA, is used to infer the likelihood of three or more distinct groups being different. It is used when you wish to find out whether three or more independent groups differ significantly from each other in the values recorded for a numerical variable. This is done by comparing the difference between the means of the groups and calculating the likelihood of the difference occurring by chance. The difference between the means of the groups is represented by the *F* value, and the likelihood of it occurring by chance by the probability (*p*).

In addition to the assumptions already outlined, ANOVA requires the data in each of the groups to have the same variance. This means that the data should have the same standard deviation. Fortunately, provided the number of cases in the largest of the groups is not more than one and a half times the number of cases in the smallest of the groups, differences in the groups' variances have little effect on the results. The way groups for ANOVA are defined is by using a categorical variable. This means that although it is similar to that described for an independent groups *t*-test, the categorical variable defines a larger number of groups (Table 6.7). ANOVA compares the differences between the means for each of the groups and calculates the probability that this difference occurred by chance. If this is low, it will be represented by a large *F* value and a probability of less than 0.05 ($p < 0.05$) and means there is a statistically significant difference.

Table 6.7 Annotated spreadsheet table with data for analysis of variance

Numerical variable records data for groups			Categorical variable divides data into three or more groups
	A	**B**	
1	**reps' sales**	**area**	
2	£27,158.00	1	
3	£45,764.00	2	
4	£86,866.00	2	
5	£24,242.00	2	
Sales by individuals are recorded in pounds	6 £53,367.00	3	
	7 £63,669.00	3	Variable 'area' is coded:
	8 £10,988.00	1	1 = North
	9 £20,393.00	2	2 = Midlands
	10 £60,459.00	3	3 = South

Pearson's product moment correlation coefficient

When analysing data you often need to establish the strength of relationship between two numerical variables and the probability that the relationship has occurred by chance. As we said earlier in this chapter (in relation to ordinal data), when a change in one variable is accompanied by a change in another variable, we say that the variables are correlated. For relationships where you know that a change in one numerical variable is accompanied by a change in another numerical variable, but it is not clear which is the independent and which is the dependent variable, you use **Pearson's product moment correlation coefficient**. This is often referred to as PMCC or Pearson's *r* (lower-case r).

Pearson's r provides a measure of the strength of the relationship between two variables and, like other correlation coefficients, the calculated statistic has a value somewhere between -1 and $+1$. As with other correlation coefficients, a correlation coefficient of (for example):

-1 means a perfect negative correlative between the two variables (as the ranks for one variable increase, the ranks of the other decrease);

0 means no correlation between the two variables;

1 means a perfect positive correlative between the two variables (as the ranks for one variable increase, the ranks of the other increase).

As you have probably noticed, this time we have not repeated values in between -1 and 0 (or 0 and 1) as we have talked about these already!

For example, if you look back to Figure 4.6, you will see a scatter graph showing the relationship between distance in miles (independent variable) and delivery time in minutes (dependent variable) for a home delivery pizza company. The data upon which this graph is based can also be used to see if, as suggested by Figure 4.6, the two variables are correlated. When we do this using statistical software such as SPSS, the software presents the data as a correlation matrix, the correlation coefficient between the named row and column variables being recorded in the cell where they intersect (Table 6.8).

If your data are collected for a sample rather than a population, you will also need to calculate the probability of your correlation having occurred by chance. In other words, you will need to calculate the probability of a sample showing a relationship as extreme as, or more extreme than that you actually observed having occurred by chance. If this probability is less than 0.05 ($p < 0.05$) then the null hypothesis of no relationship is usually rejected and you can say that the hypothesis that the relationship, represented by the correlation coefficient, is supported. Fortunately, most statistical software calculates this probability at the same time as calculating the correlation coefficient (Table 6.8).

Table 6.8   Annotated correlation matrix

Cells record the correlation coefficient between the named row variable and the named column variable			

Correlations

		distance in miles	delivery time in minutes
distance in miles	Pearson Correlation	1	.785**
	Sig. (2-tailed)		.000
	N	20	20
delivery time in minutes	Pearson Correlation	.785**	1
	Sig. (2-tailed)	.000	
	N	20	20

**. Correlation is significant at the 0.01 level (2-tailed).

Correlation coefficient between distance and time is 0.785

The probability of this correlation coefficient having occurred by chance is ≤ 0.01 (see note below table)

Correlation coefficient between a variable and itself is, inevitably, 1

Coefficient of determination

The coefficient of determination enables you to establish the strength of relationship between a numerical dependent variable and one or more numerical independent variables and the probability that the relationship has occurred by chance. As we said in Chapter 2, the dependent variable is the variable for which any change measured has happened in response to some form of manipulation of the independent variable. For relationships where you believe that a change in a dependent numerical variable is caused by a change made in another numerical independent variable, you use the **coefficient of determination**. This is often referred to as the regression coefficient or r^2 (lower-case r, squared). As you have probably guessed, this is in fact the square of Pearson's r.

Unlike correlation coefficients, the value of the coefficient of determination is always positive, lying somewhere between 0 and 1. It is often expressed as a percentage and is interpreted as the amount of variation in the dependent variable that can be explained by the independent variable. This means that, for example, a coefficient of determination of:

0   means none of the variation in the dependent variable can be explained by the independent variable;

0.3 means 30% of the variation in the dependent variable can be explained by the independent variable;

0.5 means 50% of the variation in the dependent variable can be explained by the independent variable;

0.8 means 80% of the variation in the dependent variable can be explained by the independent variable;

1 means all of the variation in the dependent variable can be explained by the independent variable.

As you have already read numerous times in this book, if your data are collected for a sample rather than a population, you will also need to calculate the probability of your coefficient of determination having occurred by chance. In other words, you will need to calculate the probability of a sample showing a relationship as extreme as, or more extreme than that you actually observed having occurred by chance. If this probability is less than 0.05 ($p < 0.05$) then the null hypothesis of no relationship is usually rejected and you can say that the hypothesis that the relationship, represented by the coefficient of determination, is supported. As you know by now, most statistical software calculates this probability at the same time as calculating the correlation coefficient.

Final comments

As will be obvious to you, we have only skated the surface of the statistical tests you can use for quantitative research. This is why we have insisted that you use the period of time when you are designing your questionnaire or interview schedule to clarify for yourself the kind of tests that will be the most appropriate to give you the findings that you are aiming for.

We hope that this chapter has interested you and has given you a taste of the fascinating things you can do with statistics, so that you will be inclined to go further into the topic.

Chapter 7

What next?

Where you are now

What we have done in this book is to skim over the surface of statistics in order to give you a feel for the main areas that will be of interest to you when you are undertaking your project. If you have read to this point, then you should now have a grasp of the concepts and terminology of basic statistics. This will help you in three ways. You are now more likely to:

- read reports, journal articles, newspaper articles and books with the ability to see the point of the statistics they might contain, and, more importantly, to understand the descriptions of the various statistical tests that the author used to analyse the data and produce findings from them;
- present your own research so that the reader is more likely to accept your findings because they are based on a robust analysis;
- find it easier to understand other statistics books which tackle the topic in more detail.

What you now know

Having read the book, the list of what you now know is lengthy:

1. Statistics can help you to draw conclusions within boundaries set by your sample, your data collection techniques or your analysis procedures.
2. You can quantify your findings.

3. You can make generalisations from what you know from your data (your sample) to a wider group (the population).

4. You can begin to understand your data by presenting it as tables and graphs.

5. Different graphs are better for illustrating different aspects of your data, and your choice of graph will also depend upon the type of data.

6. It is helpful to begin your statistical analysis by describing your data.

7. You can describe the location (central tendency) and, where appropriate, the dispersion (spread) of data variables using statistics appropriate to the level of measurement of your data.

8. You can use index numbers to describe the relative change in a series of data values over time for a particular variable.

9. There is a test (chi-square) that will help you decide whether the pattern you observe in your data is significantly different from that which would have been expected by chance, when you are looking at categorical rather than quantitative data variables.

10. You can use different correlation statistics to measure the strength of a relationship between two ordinal variables (Kendall's or Spearman's) or between two numerical variables (Pearson's).

11. You need to bear in mind that correlations don't measure the strength of a cause-and-effect relationship, and that the fact that there is a relationship between two variables doesn't mean that one caused the other.

12. You use alternative statistical tests to infer the likelihood that two or more groups are different, depending upon whether the data are in pairs (paired t-test or independent groups t-test) and the number of groups (independent groups t-test or analysis of variance).

13. You can use the coefficient of determination to measure the proportion of a dependent variable explained by an independent variable.

14. You can make sensible inferences about a population, based on the statistics from the sample.

15. Something which is statistically significant may not be of importance in any practical sense, and so you won't confuse the two.

16. Statistical techniques can be hijacked and can be used to enhance biased views or to 'prove' a pet theory or viewpoint, and so you need to take care with choosing and using your own statistical test.

17. Statistics never prove anything completely. The best that the techniques can do is provide very strong support for your assumptions, inferences and conclusions, but they will never give you total, absolute proof.

So, what next?

That depends on where you want to go. If this book has shown you that statistics is both interesting and useful, you might want to go deeper into the topic. If you are a minimalist as far as statistics are concerned, then you now know which statistical tests will enable you to 'get by' and produce a convincing project. Hopefully, you will also know when someone is trying to deceive you by quoting statistics that do not appear sensible. Whichever route you select, we wish you enjoyment in your discoveries, and success in your research endeavours.

Appendix 1

Asking questions and types of data

This appendix describes different questions and statements you might use in your primary data collection, and the types of data associated with them.

Asking questions

Clearly, the questions you have asked will affect the tests you can run on the data which you have gathered when asking those questions. In Table A1.1 we have put together questions from an assortment of management disciplines as examples of the kinds of things you might want to ask, giving the relevant variables and the types of data that apply to them.

Table A1.1   Research questions, variables and types of data

Area of research interest	Research question	Variable of interest	Type of data
Accounting	Which budget-setting techniques has the firm used over the past 10 years?	Relative performance of different budget-setting techniques	Ordinal

Finance	How has the firm's share price behaved over the past decade?	Prices of shares over the decade	Ratio
Information systems	Has the introduction of new systems improved the output of individual administrative staff?	Output in the form of the volume of work undertaken before and after introduction	Ratio
Management	Is the average age of the employees that the firm has made redundant higher than the age of the employees who remain?	Ages of employees in both groups	Ratio
Marketing	Does the use of different ethnic groups in a television advert increase product preference among consumers from those ethnic groups?	Relative preference for one product over another by group	Ordinal

Table A1.2 provides a reminder of the different individual questions you could ask, defining them, and giving examples.

Table A1.2 Types of questions

Type	Definition and example
Number	The response is a number, giving the amount of some characteristic.

In which year did you join the company?
On what date were you made redundant?
In what year were you born? |

Category	The response is one of a given set of categories, and the interviewee or questionnaire respondent can only fit into one.
	In which age group do you belong? 20–29 ☐ 30–39 ☐ 40–49 ☐ 50–59 ☐
	Have you studied, or are you now studying, for a professional qualification? Yes, in the past ☐ Yes, currently ☐ Never ☐
List	The response is to a list of items offered, any of which may be selected.
	Which of the following do you think applies to your department? Tick all boxes that apply. Is efficient ☐ Has lost its way ☐ Manager is dynamic ☐ Manager is ineffective ☐ Colleagues are supportive ☐ Colleagues are competitive ☐
Ranking	Responses are placed in rank order. Ranking is most often used for attitudes, qualities or characteristics.
	What do you think were the reasons behind the company's current change initiative? Please rank them in order of importance, numbering the most important 1, the next 2 and so on. Drive for efficiency ☐ To remedy current problems ☐ Power issues ☐ Current management fad ☐ Change for change's sake ☐ Management politics ☐
Scale	The response gives the strength of feeling or of attitudes.
	To what extent do you think your company is ethical? Very ethical ☐ Somewhat ethical ☐ Ethical ☐ Somewhat unethical ☐ Very unethical ☐

Open-ended	The response is a word, phrase or even an extended comment. The intention is to give interviewees or respondents to give their views on the topic being researched.
	Please provide your views on the company's redundancy policy in the space below.
	Please state your reasons for disagreeing with the above question.

Table A1.3 presents an example of questions, the types of data that they generate and the way in which they could be coded.

Table A1.3   Examples of questions, type of data and coding

Question	Type of data	Coding
Are you? (Circle your answer) Male Female	Nominal	Male = 1, Female = 2
What is your age in years?	Ratio	
In which age group would you place yourself? (e.g. 20–29, 30–39)	Ordinal	20–29 = 1 30–39 = 2 etc.
What is your work grade? Manager ☐ Deputy Manager ☐ Administrator ☐ Senior clerk ☐ Junior clerk ☐	Ordinal	Manager = 5 Deputy Manager = 4 Administrator = 3 Senior clerk = 2 Junior clerk = 1
Are you employed full-time or part-time? Full time ☐ Part time ☐	Ordinal	Full-time = 1 Part-time = 2

State the number of hours and minutes you work each week Marketing ☐ Accounting ☐ HR ☐	Ratio	
In which department do you work?	Nominal	Marketing = 1 Accounting = 2 HR = 3 No response = 9
How many people work in your department?	Ratio	
Circle the number which best describes how satisfied you are with the quality of service you have received. completely dissatisfied 1 dissatisfied 2 neutral 3 satisfied 4 Completely satisfied 5	Ordinal	1 = completely dissatisfied 2 = dissatisfied 3 = neutral 4 = satisfied 5 = completely satisfied

If you have used a questionnaire, it may be helpful remind you briefly of the types of questions and the rating scales available to you when you design your questionnaire, and to illustrate, again, how intertwined questionnaire design and measurement are. Table A1.4 presents examples of rating questions for different scales, highlighting the different types of data collected.

Table A1.4   Scales, types of data and example questions

Scale	Type of data	Example question
Simple category, dichotomous	Nominal	I own a mobile phone ☐ $_1$ Yes ☐ $_2$ No
Multiple choice, single response	Nominal	If you had to choose one newspaper to read on Sundays, which from the list below would you select? Tick only one. ☐ $_1$ *The Sunday Record* ☐ $_2$ *Sunday Journal* ☐ $_3$ *News on Sunday* ☐ $_4$ *The Review on Sunday*
Multiple choice, multipleresponse	Nominal	Please tick all of the papers below that you read on Sundays. ☐ *The Sunday Record* ☐ *Sunday Journal* ☐ *News on Sunday* ☐ *The Review on Sunday* ☐ Other (please describe) ....
Rating	Ordinal	'SearchHere' is easier to use than 'FindItOut' as an Internet search engine. Please indicate how strongly you agree or disagree with this statement. strongly agree agree neutral disagree strongly disagree 1 2 3 4 5

Ranking	Ordinal	Please write your ranking of the items below, using 1 for most important, 2 for next most important, and so on. Fast service ☐ Reliable service ☐ Cheap prices ☐ Wide product range ☐ 30-day credit ☐ Returns policy ☐
Numerical	Interval	On a scale of 1 to 10, please write the appropriate number against the statements below extremely extremely unfavourable 1 2 3 4 5 6 7 8 9 10 favourable My line manager cares about my welfare ……… My line manager is strongly directive …….
Multiple rating list	Interval	Please indicate on a scale of 5 to 1 how important or unimportant you consider each characteristic of this product's supplier important unimportant Fast 5 4 3 2 1 Reliable 5 4 3 2 1 Good value 5 4 3 2 1

Before choosing a statistical test

The kinds of questions you need to ask yourself before you choose a particular test are as follows:

- What is the research question I am trying to answer?

- What are the characteristics of the sample? For instance, is the sample type random, snowball, convenience, …?

- What type(s) of data do I have? For instance, are the data categorical or numerical, discrete, dichotomous or continuous, nominal, ordinal, interval or ratio?

- How many data variables are there?

- How many groups are there?

- Are the data distributed normally?

- If the data are not distributed normally, will this affect the statistic I want to use?

- Are the samples (groups) independent?

In addition, if you intend to make inferences about a population from your sample, the inferences you will be able to make will depend upon answers to questions such as these:

- Are the data representative of the population?

- Are the groups different?

- Is there a relationship between the variables?

Which test to choose

To select the right test, ask yourself three questions:

- What type(s) of data have been collected?

- What are the measurement properties of these data?

- What do I wish to find out?

A reminder of the types of variables which can be measured at the levels shown is given in Table A1.5.

Table A1.5   Examples of measurement properties for types of
quantitative data

Type	Discrete (names)	Discrete (numbers)	Continuous
Nominal	Age	Street numbers	—
Ordinal	Grade at work	Class of travel (1st, 2nd)	—
Interval	—	IQ scores	Temperature
Ratio	—	Department size	Weight

Choosing between non-parametric and parametric statistics

Whether to choose a non-parametric or a parametric statistical test is in part a matter of judgement. Although it is generally agreed that parametric statistics are designed for numerical (interval and ratio) data which are normally distributed, it is worth remembering the following:

- Some statisticians use non-parametric tests for all data types where the sample size is small (below 30).
- If you are replicating analyses undertaken by another researcher, it might be appropriate to select your test on the basis of what she or he used.
- In general, both non-parametric tests and parametric tests can be used with numerical data as long as the sample is large. Although it is impossible to say how 'large' is 'large enough', 30 is often used, provided the data are normally distributed.

Appendix 2

Useful statistical software

Two software packages which are widely used to do statistical tests are discussed, beginning with the spreadsheet Excel, and then moving on to the more advanced statistical analysis software SPSS.

While this book was written to provide you with the basic or introductory statistical knowledge that you need in order to undertake the analysis of your data so that you can understand and interpret them, it seemed sensible to tell you about two of the most frequently used statistical software packages that will draw your graphs, create your tables and calculate your statistics. These can be grouped into two types of packages: spreadsheets such as Excel, and more advanced statistical analysis software such as SPSS.

Obviously, you will need to learn how to enter your data. This is relatively simple, with most statistical software packages accepting data as a matrix in which each row represents a separate case and each column represents a separate variable (Figures A2.1 and A2.2). Once you have done this and have decided which statistical tests you wish to use, then the packages will run the analyses you ask for, and display the results in tables and graphs almost instantaneously.

The next bit of learning you will need to undertake is to understand what the various output tables are showing you in order to interpret the results, but there are books that will help you with this as well as the online help associated with the software.

Spreadsheets: Excel

You have almost certainly been introduced to Excel already. While Excel is a software program designed to help you evaluate and

Figure A2.1   Annotated extract from an Excel data matrix

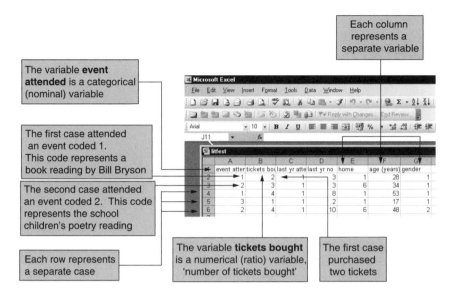

Each column represents a separate variable

The variable **event attended** is a categorical (nominal) variable

The first case attended an event coded 1. This code represents a book reading by Bill Bryson

The second case attended an event coded 2. This code represents the school children's poetry reading

Each row represents a separate case

The variable **tickets bought** is a numerical (ratio) variable, 'number of tickets bought'

The first case purchased two tickets

Figure A2.2   Annotated extract from an SPSS data matrix

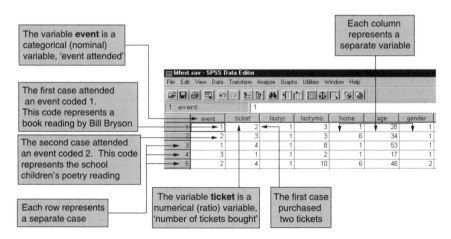

Each column represents a separate variable

The variable **event** is a categorical (nominal) variable, 'event attended'

The first case attended an event coded 1. This code represents a book reading by Bill Bryson

The second case attended an event coded 2. This code represents the school children's poetry reading

Each row represents a separate case

The variable **ticket** is a numerical (ratio) variable, 'number of tickets bought'

The first case purchased two tickets

present data in spreadsheets, it is far more than that. For example, tables and graphs can be constructed by selecting the 'Data' menu and then clicking on 'PivotTable and PivotChart Report ...', and graphs can also be drawn using the Chart Wizard. More frequently used descriptive statistics can be calculated by selecting 'Function' from the 'Insert' menu, a wide variety of other statistics being available through the 'Tools' menu. By selecting the 'Tools' menu, clicking on 'Add-Ins ...', selecting the 'Analysis ToolPak' and clicking on 'OK', you will then see a new 'Tools' menu item called 'Data Analysis ...'. Within this you will find a list of additional statistical tests that you can use. These include many of the statistical tests we have discussed in this book.

Excel runs statistical tests on data that are either entered into a worksheet manually or imported as a data matrix from text files or databases. You then select the analysis procedure you intend to use, select the variables that you wish to analyse and run the test. You can also use Excel's charting options to produce a variety of charts and graphs to illustrate your findings, such as those outlined in Chapter 4.

Statistical analysis software: SPSS

SPSS provides a tutorial that will help you to teach yourself how to use the package. Analysing data using SPSS is straightforward provided you know which statistics you want to use. Obviously you need to enter your data, either by typing them in as a data matrix, using the SPSS Data Editor's 'Data View' window, or importing them directly from another software package (e.g. a spreadsheet such as Excel). Subsequently, you decide on the graph you wish to draw and select it from the 'Graphs' menu, or the analysis procedure you wish to use and select it from the 'Analyze' menu.

SPSS allows you to label your variables and, for categorical data, your data values using the SPSS Data Editor's 'Variable View' window. It also allows you to transform your data, for example by recoding variables or computing new variables. The software can create cross-tabulations and calculate a far wider variety of statistical tests than Excel, ranging from frequency tables to very sophisticated multivariate analyses. These are known as 'procedures'. After you have chosen your procedure, you need to select the variables you wish to analyse. To run the analysis, all you need to do is to point and click.

You need to learn how to interpret the way in which the results of your analysis are presented as output in the SPSS Viewer window (we have included a few examples in this book), but once you have done this, you come to the interesting bit, and the point of the whole process – examining and interpreting your results.

Appendix 3

An alphabet of statistics

In the table below, the first column gives the letters in the Latin or Greek alphabet, and the second column gives their meaning. Within this table, we have only included those used in this book.

letter(s)	meaning
ANOVA	Analysis of variance
f	Frequency – the number of times a given value occurs
F	F value, calculated when conducting an analysis of variance
H_0	Null hypothesis
H_1	Alternative hypothesis
H_a	Alternative hypothesis
n	(lower case) The number of cases in a sample
N	(upper case) The number of cases in a population
p	Probability value (e.g. $p < 0.05$)
PMCC	Pearson's product moment correlation coefficient
r	Pearson's product moment correlation coefficient
r_S	Spearman's rank correlation coefficient
r^2	Coefficient of determination (regression coefficient)
s	Standard deviation of a sample
t	t value, calculated when conducting a t-test
x	A collective symbol meaning all the individual values, often used to represent an independent variable
$\bar{x}$ (x-bar)	(Arithmetic) mean of a sample
y	An alternative symbol to x, often used to represent the dependent variable

μ (mu)	Mean of a population
ρ (rho)	Spearman's rank correlation coefficient
σ (sigma)	Standard deviation of a population
τ (tau)	Kendall's rank correlation coefficient
χ^2 (chi-square)	chi-square test

Glossary

A

Alphabetical variable: A variable where the data are letters, often words.

Alphanumeric variable: A variable where the data are a combination of letters and numbers.

Alternative hypothesis: *See* hypothesis.

Analysis of variance (ANOVA): A statistic to infer association between three or more distinct groups, by stating the likelihood of any difference between the values for a numerical variable for each of the groups (defined by a separate variable) having occurred by chance alone.

Arithmetic mean: *See* mean.

Assumption: A statement about the data which needs to be true if a statistic is to be reliable. Most parametric statistical techniques require that certain assumptions can be made about the data.

Attribute: A categorical variable or constant.

Average index: A series of numbers calculated to describe the average relative change in a series of values for a number of numerical variables over time.

B

Bar chart: A graph normally used to show the frequency of occurrence and emphasise the highest and lowest categories for one categorical data variable, in which the length (or height) of each bar represents the responses to one category. Can also be used to show the trends for a variable over time.

Base period: The period with which a comparison is being made such as when using an index number. *See:* simple index number, average index, weighted average index.

Bias: Any systematic error resulting from the data collection procedures used.

Bimodal distribution: A distribution which has two modes.

C

Cardinal numbers: The numbers 1, 2, 3 and so on.

Case: An individual item in a population or sample.

Categorical variable: A variable where the data are grouped into categories (sets) or placed in rank order.

Categories: partitioned subsets of a data variable, usually represented by codes.

Categorisation: The process of using rules to partition data into categories.

Census: In statistics, conducting a census refers to collecting data from an entire population.

Chi-square test: A statistical test to infer association between two categorical variables, by stating whether there is a statistically significant difference between the observed distribution pattern of data in a two-way table (in which the categories of one of the variables form the rows and the categories of the other variable form the columns) and that which would have been expected by chance. *See also:* one-sample chi-square test.

Closed question: Question used to constrain the person answering to a limited number of predetermined responses.

Code: A number or other character assigned to a specific response.

Code book: A list of variables in a study containing the question number, variable name, variable label, code and associated label.

Coding: Assigning numbers or other characters to answers so that responses can be grouped into classes or categories.

Coefficient of determination: A statistic to infer association between a dependent and an independent numerical variable, by assessing the strength of a cause-and-effect relationship through the level of agreement between the two sets of values and its statistical significance; that is, the likelihood of this having occurred by chance alone. Also termed: regression coefficient.

Coefficient of multiple determination: A statistic to infer association between a dependent numerical variable and two or more independent numerical variables, by assessing the strength of a cause-and-effect relationship through the level of agreement between the values of the dependent and independent variables and its statistical significance; that is, the likelihood of this having occurred by chance alone. Also termed: multiple regression coefficient.

Confidence interval: The accuracy of a prediction or estimate of a population made from a sample; usually expressed as plus or minus a percentage.

Confidence level: The degree of certainty that a prediction or estimate about a population made from a sample is accurate; usually expressed as a percentage.

Constant: An attribute, trait or characteristic which only has one value. In other words, not a variable.

Contingency table: *See* cross-tabulation.

Continuous variable: A variable where the data can take on certain values, sometimes within a finite range.

Correlation: The extent to which a change in one variable is accompanied by a change in another variable.

Correlation coefficient: A statistic which measure of the strength of the relationship between two variables, in other words, the extent to which the two variables are associated. Often called a measure of association, the statistic's value ranges from −1.0 to +1.0.

Cross-tabulation: A table summarising the number of cases in each category for two or more variables. Also known as a contingency table.

.

D

Data: Facts that have been obtained and subsequently recorded. Remember that 'data' are plural, and that one item of data is a datum.

Data presentation: the use of tables and graphs to illustrate your data.

Data set: A collection of data items, such as the answers given by respondents to all the questions in a questionnaire.

Data type: *See* nominal, ordinal, interval, ratio variable.

Dependent variable: The variable that is measured in response to manipulation of the independent variable.

Descriptive statistics: Statistics that describe quantitative data. Often contrasted with inferential statistics, which are used to make inferences about a population based on information about a sample drawn from that population.

Dichotomous variable: A categorical variable that has only two categories, such as male/female, pass/fail, yes/no.

Discrete variable: A variable where the data can only take on certain values which are clearly separated from one another.

Dispersion: *See* measure of dispersion

E

Empirical rule: For a normal distribution, 68% of the data will fall within one standard deviation of the mean and 95% of the data will fall within two standard deviations of the mean.

F

Fisher's exact test: A statistical test to infer association between two nominal variables, by stating whether there is a statistically significant difference between the observed distribution pattern of data in a two-way table (in which the categories of one of the variables form two rows and the categories of the other variable form two columns) and that which would have been expected by chance.

Frequency: The number of times a particular type of event occurs or the number of individuals in a given category.

Frequency distribution: *See* frequency table.

Frequency polygon: A line graph normally used to show frequency of occurrence and emphasise the highest and lowest categories for one variable or to show the distribution of categories for one variable (frequencies are normally displayed vertically and categories horizontally, and the data values will need to be grouped into categories). *See also* line graph.

Frequency table: A table summarising the number of cases in each category for a variable.

H

Histogram: A graph normally used to show the frequency of occurrence and emphasise the highest and lowest categories for one numerical data variable in which the area of each bar represents the responses to one category.

Hypothesis: A statement of, or a conjecture about, the relationship or difference between two or more variables that you intend to study. If testable, hypotheses are thought of as predictions, which, if confirmed, will support a theory.

Hypothesis testing: Assessing the validity or otherwise of a hypothesis when you have collected data from a sample by calculating the probability that the data collected reveal true patterns, such as a relationship between two variables, in the population from which they were drawn, rather than these patterns having occurred by chance alone.

I

Independent groups *t*-test: A statistic to infer association between two distinct groups, by stating the likelihood of any differences between the values for a numerical variable for each of the two groups (defined by a separate variable) having occurred by chance alone.

Independent variable: The variable manipulated (altered or changed) to find out its effect on the dependent variable.

Index numbers: *See* simple index number, average index, weighted average index.

Inductive: Reasoning that begins with observation and then moves from observation of particulars to the development of general hypotheses.

Inferential statistics: Statistics that allow you to draw conclusions or make inferences about a population by analysing data collected from a sample drawn from that population.

Inter-quartile range: A statistic that describes a data variable by measuring the dispersion (spread), stating the difference within the middle 50% of ranked data values for one variable.

Interval scale: A measurement scale in which numbers can be used to calculate the precise numeric distance between any two values, but not the relative difference.

Interval variable: A numerical variable where the difference between any two values in the data set can stated numerically, but not the relative difference.

K

Kendall's rank correlation coefficient: A statistical test to infer association between two ordinal variables, by assessing the strength of a relationship through the level of agreement between the two sets of rankings (being more appropriate if a variable contains tied ranks) and its statistical significance; that is, the likelihood of it having occurred by chance.

Kolmogorov–Smirnov test: A statistical test to infer association between two ordinal variables, by stating whether the differences in the location and shape of the distribution of the two groups are statistically significant; that is, significantly different from what would have been expected by chance.

Kurtosis: A statistic that describes a data variable by measuring the dispersion (spread), stating how the pointedness or flatness of the shape of the distribution of the data values for a variable differs from the normal distribution.

L

Likelihood: The probability of what has been inferred about a population from a sample being true.

Line graph: A graph normally used to show the trend for one numerical data variable over time in which each data point on the line represents the amount at a particular time.

Lower quartile: the value located 25% of the way through the ranked data values for a variable when starting with the lowest value.

M

Mann–Whitney U-test: A statistical test to infer association between two ordinal variables, by stating whether the difference between the location of the two groups is statistically significant; that is, signifi-cantly different from that which would have been expected by chance.

Mean (arithmetic mean): A statistic that describes a data variable by measuring the location (central tendency), stating the average data value of the set of data values for one variable.

Measurement: The assignment of numbers to the attributes, traits or characteristics on which cases differ.

Measurement scale: The way in which the data in a variable are measured. *See* interval scale, nominal scale, ordinal scale, ratio scale.

Measure of association: A measure that infers the strength of a relationship between two or more variables.

Measure of central tendency: *See* measure of location.

Measure of dispersion: A measure that describes the spread or variability of data values for a numeric variable. Depending upon the type of data, the more common measures of dispersion are the range, inter-quartile range and standard deviation.

Measure of location: A measure that describes what is common, middling or average for a variable. Depending upon the type of data, the more common measures are the mode, median and mean.

Measure of spread: *See* measure of dispersion.

Median: A statistic that describes a data variable by measuring the location (central tendency), stating the middle data value of the set of ranked data values for one variable.

Mid spread: *See* inter-quartile range.

Mode: A statistic that describes a data variable by measuring the location (central tendency), stating the most frequently occurring category or categories for one variable.

Multimodal distribution: A distribution which has multiple (more than two) modes.

Multiple bar chart: A graph normally used to compare the frequency of occurrence and emphasise the highest and lowest categories for two or more categorical data variables in which the length (or height) of each bar represents the responses to one category. Can also be used to compare the trends for two or more variables over time.

Multiple line graph: A graph normally used to compare the trend for two or more numerical data variables over time in which each data point on a line represents the amount at a particular time.

Multiple regression coefficient: *See* coefficient of multiple determination.

Mutually exclusive: Conditions, states, events or responses that cannot be placed in more than one category, for example, male and female, yes and no.

N

Negative number: A number that is less than zero. Written with a minus sign in front of it – for instance, –10° is 10 degrees below zero.

Negatively skewed: A distribution in which the tail stretches towards the smaller values.

Nominal scale: A measurement scale in which codes are used to represent labels for each category, but have no order or value.

Nominal variable: A categorical variable where the data are grouped into descriptive categories by name which, although they cannot be ranked, count the number of occurrences.

Non-parametric statistics: Statistical tests of significance to infer differences and relationships between categorical data variables.

Non-probability sample: A sample where the probability of each case being selected is not known and there is no sampling frame.

Non-random sample: *See* non-probability sample.

Normal distribution: A distribution in which the data values for a variable are clustered around the mean in a symmetrical pattern forming a bell-shaped frequency curve. In a normal distribution, the mean, median, and mode are all the same.

Null hypothesis: A statement, or a conjecture, stating that there is no significant relationship or difference between two or more variables that you intend to study.

Numerical variable: A variable where the data are numbers, being either counts or measures.

O

One-sample chi-square test: A statistic that describes a data variable by measuring the dispersion (spread), stating whether there is a significant difference between the observed distribution pattern of data between the categories and that which would have been expected had there been no pattern.

Open question: Question allowing the person answering to respond in their own words, often requiring a narrative response.

Ordinal numbers: Numbers describing a ranking or position such as 1st, 2nd, 3rd and so on.

Ordinal scale: A measurement scale in which numbers represent the order or rank for each case and consequently the relative position.

Ordinal variable: A categorical variable where the relative position of each case within the data set is known, giving a definite order or rank.

Outlier: A data value that is extremely high or extremely low compared with the rest of the data for a variable.

P

Paired *t*-test: A statistic to infer association between two distinct groups (where the numerical data values are in pairs, one from each group) by stating the likelihood of any difference between the paired values from the two groups (each group's values being contained in a separate variable) having occurred by chance alone.

Parameter: a numerical measure that describes some characteristic of the population.

Parametric statistics: Statistical tests of significance to infer differences and relationships between numerical data variables.

Pearson's product moment correlation coefficient (PMCC): A statistic to infer association between a dependent and an independent numerical variable, by assessing the strength of a relationship through the level of agreement between the two sets of values and its statistical significance; that is, the likelihood of this having occurred by chance alone.

Pie chart: A graph normally used to show the proportions in each category for one categorical data variable in which each slice of the pie represents the responses to one category.

Population: The complete set of things that is of interest to you in its own right, rather than because they are representative of something larger. Also termed: universe.

Positively skewed: A distribution in which the tail stretches towards the larger values.

Practical significance: A research finding which reveals something meaningful about the object of study. Also termed: substantive significance.

Primary data: Data collected specifically for your research project.

Probability: The likelihood that a particular finding or relationship between variables will have occurred (by chance) when inferring about a population from a sample.

Probability sample: A sample in which each case in the population has a known probability of being selected.

Q

Quartiles: Divisions of the ranked data values for a variable into four groups of equal size using the lower quartile, median and upper quartile.

Quota sample: A sample based on the idea that it will represent the population if the variability for certain known quota variables is the same as in the population.

R

Range: A statistic that describes a data variable by measuring the dispersion (spread), stating the difference between the highest and lowest ranked data values for one variable.

Ratio scale: A measurement scale in which numbers can be used to calculate the precise numeric distance and relative difference or ratio between any two values in the data.

Ratio variable: A numerical variable where the relative difference, or ratio, between any two values in the data can be calculated.

Regression coefficient: *See* coefficient of determination.

Regression equation (1): An equation to infer a dependent numerical variable's values by prediction from one or more independent numerical variable's values and its statistical significance; that is, the likelihood of this having occurred by chance alone. (**2**): An equation to infer the long-term or secular trend of a series of data values for a dependent numerical variable over time and its statistical significance; that is, the likelihood of this having occurred by chance alone.

Representative sample: A sample that represents the population from which it was drawn. A representative sample can be used to make inferences about the population. *See also* probability sample.

Representativeness: The extent to which a study's results can be generalised to other situations or settings.

S

Sample: A group of cases selected, usually from the complete set or population. The intention is that, in studying this smaller group, you will reveal things about the population.

Sampling frame: A complete list of the total population from which a probability sample can subsequently be selected.

Scale: The combination of the scored responses from a number of scale items to create a measure for a concept such as trust.

Scale item: One of a number of rating questions combined to create a scale.

Scatter graph: A graph normally used to show the relationship between two numerical data variables in which each data point represents the relationship between the two variables for a case.

Secondary data: Data that you use that were originally collected for some purpose other than the research project for which they are now being used.

Significance testing: *See* statistical significance testing.

Simple index numbers: A series of numbers calculated to describe the relative change in a series of values for a numerical variable over time.

Skewness: A statistic that describes a data variable by measuring the dispersion (spread), stating how the shape of the distribution of the data values for a variable deviates from a symmetrical (normal) distribution. *See also* positively skewed, negatively skewed.

Spearman's rank correlation coefficient: A statistical test to infer association between two ordinal variables, by assessing the strength of a relationship through the level of agreement between the two sets of rankings (being more appropriate if a variable does not contain tied ranks) and its statistical significance; that is, the likelihood of it having occurred by chance.

Spread: *See* dispersion.

Standard deviation: A statistic that describes a data variable by measuring the dispersion (spread), stating the extent the data values for one variable are spread around its mean using the same units as those in which the data were recorded.

Statistic: A numerical measure that describes some characteristic of the sample.

Statistical association: *See* measure of association.

Statistical significance testing: Testing the probability of a pattern such as a relationship between two variables, defined by a hypothesis, occurring by chance alone. Remember that statistical significance doesn't necessarily imply practical significance – for instance, you may have statistically significant results that are actually of no importance or have no relevance in practical terms.

Summary statistics: *See* descriptive statistics.

T

Tail: The part of a skewed distribution that stretches out to one side or the other.

Test statistic: A statistic used to test a finding or hypothesis about a sample for statistical significance.

True zero: When the value represented by zero is the absence of the thing being measured and shows the point where measurement begins.

***t*-test:** *See* independent groups *t*-test, paired *t*-test.

Two-sample chi-square test: *See* chi-square test.

Type I error: An error made by rejecting a null hypothesis when, in reality, it is correct. This means, in effect, incorrectly accepting a hypothesis.

Type II error: An error made by failing to reject a null hypothesis when, in reality, it is incorrect. This means, in effect, incorrectly rejecting a hypothesis.

Type of data: *See* nominal, ordinal, interval, ratio variable.

U

Universe: See population.

Upper quartile: the value located 75% of the way through the ranked data values for a variable when starting with the lowest value.

V

Variable: Any attribute, trait or characteristic that can have more than one value.

Variance: A statistic that describes a data variable by measuring the dispersion (spread), stating the extent to which the data values for one variable are spread around its mean, but in the square of the units in which the data were recorded.

W

Weighted average index: A series of numbers calculated to describe the average relative change in a series of values for a number of numerical variables over time, individual variables within the index being weighted according to their relative importance.

INDEX

Page numbers for figures have suffix **f,** those for tables have suffix **t**

Business Research Methods 2/e

Boris Blumberg

Business Research Methods second edition presents a balanced and comprehensive account of business research that is engaging, rigorous and up-to-date. The text explores all the topics involved in the research process, both theoretical and practical, in an accessible manner. This edition also boasts a number of new features and examples to thoroughly explain and illustrate the concepts, processes and practices of good business research.

NEW features include:

- New chapter on Case Studies and Qualitative Interviews
- Running case study
- Example of a good proposal
- Up-to-date coverage

New design

This edition also includes a free CD-Rom that contains five additional chapters. These cover the statistical background to business research with a chapter on each of the following: Data Preparation, Displaying and Preparing Data, Hypothesis Testing, Measure of Association and Multivariate Analysis.

An Online Learning Centre accompanies Business Research Methods second edition. The site includes extensive resources for both lecturers and students.

Contents: Part I Essentials of Research – The nature of business and management research – Research process and proposal – Literature review – Research Ethics – **Part II Research Approaches** – Quantitative and qualitative research – Sampling strategies: from one case to the whole population – Survey Research – Secondary data, archival sources and content analysis – Observational, action and ethnographic research – Case Studies and Qualitative Interviews (NEW!) – Experiments – **Part III Research Instruments** – Measurements and scales – Field work: questionnaire and responses – Writing and presenting research outcomes – **Part IV Statistical background (on CD-ROM)** – Data preparation and description – Exploring, displaying and examining data – Hypothesis testing – Measure of association – Multivariate analysis: an overview

2008 770pp

ISBN 978-0-077-11745-0   Paperback

Business Research Methods, with Student DVD, 10/e
Donald R. Cooper and Pamela S. Schindler

In this comprehensively revised 10th edition, Students and instructors will find thorough coverage of business research topics – including the best coverage of questionnaire design – backed by solid theory. Managerial decision making is the underlying theme, and topics and applications are presented and organized in a manner that allows students to thoroughly understand business research topics and functions. Consequently, the structure of the text encourages and supports completion of an in-depth business research project during the semester.

New to this edition

- Material was reorganized to match the way instructors teach and to address problems they face in teaching research methods.
- Research terminology is now addressed, along with the building blocks of the scientific method, in order to discuss how to correctly analyze research problems.
- Examples on Experimentation were revised to include more functional areas of business, and more complex materials (designs and test markets) were placed in a chapter appendix.
- New video material offers the only video on a Metaphorical Elicitation Technique 'MET' interview, as well as video material and video cases on the text-enclosed DVD.

Features

- A business focus has been integrated throughout the text. Students are presented with a 'real-world' approach to business research topics and how they are used in business.
- The Online Learning Center includes sample proposals, sample instruments, sample research reports, and more.
- SPSS software packaging option: The student software version will allow students an opportunity to gain experience with this tool and apply it to the applications in the text.

Content: Part I: Introduction to Business Research – Research in Business – Ethics in Business Research – Thinking Like a Researcher – The Research Process: An Overview – Clarifying the Research Question through Secondary Data and Exploration – Appendix 5A: Bibliographic Database Searches – Appendix 5B: Advanced Searches – **Part II: The Design of Business Research** – Research Design: An Overview – Qualitative Research – Observation Studies – Surveys – Experiments – Appendix 10A: Complex Experimental Designs – Appendix 10B: Test Markets – **Part III: The Sources and Collection of Data** – Measurement – Measurement Scales – Questionnaires and Instruments – Appendix 13A: Crafting Effective Measurement Questions – Appendix 13B: Pretesting Options and Discoveries – Sampling – Appendix 14A: Determining Sample Size – **Part IV: Insights from Findings: Analysis and Presentation of Data** – Data Preparation and Description – Appendix 15A: Describing Data Statistically – Exploring, Displaying, and Examining Data – Hypothesis Testing – Measures of Association – Multivariate Analysis: An Overview – Presenting Results: Oral and Written Reports Case Abstracts – Appendices: A. Business Research Requests and Proposals (with Sample RFP) – B. Focus Group Discussion Guide – C. Nonparametric Significance Tests – D. Selected Statistical Tables – References and Readings – Glossary of Key Terms

February 2008

ISBN: 978-0-071-26333-7 Paperback

ISBN: 978-0-077-22487-5 Hardback

Quantitative Data Analysis using SPSS: An Introduction for Health and Social Sciences

Pete Greasley

This accessible book is essential reading for those looking for a short and simple guide to basic data analysis. Written for the complete beginner, the book is the ideal companion when undertaking quantitative data analysis for the first time using SPSS.

The book uses a simple example of quantitative data analysis that would be typical to the health field to take you through the process of data analysis step by step. The example used is a doctor who conducts a questionnaire survey of 30 patients to assess a specific service. The data from these questionnaires is given to you for analysis, and the book leads you through the process required to analyse this data.

Handy screenshots illustrate each step of the process so you can try out the analysis for yourself, and apply it to your own research with ease.

Topics covered include:

- Questionnaires and how to analyse them
- Coding the data for SPSS, setting up an SPSS database and entering the data
- Descriptive statistics and illustrating the data using graphs
- Cross-tabulation and the Chi-square statistic
- Correlation: examining relationships between interval data
- Examining differences between two sets of scores

Reporting the results and presenting the data

Quantitative Data Analysis Using SPSS is helpful for any students in health and social sciences with little or no experience of quantitative data analysis and statistics.

Contents: Introduction – A questionnaire and what to do with it: types of data and relevant analyses – Coding the data for SPSS, setting up an SPSS database and entering the data – Descriptive statistics: Frequencies, measures of central tendency and illustrating the data using graphs – Cross-tabulation and the Chi-square statistic – Correlation: Examining relationships between interval data – Examining differences between two sets of scores – Reporting the results and presenting the data – Conclusion – References – Answers to the Quiz and Exercises – Glossary

2007 160pp

ISBN: 978-0-335-22305-3   Paperback

ISBN: 978-0-335-22306-0   Hardback

SPSS Survival Manual: A Step by Step Guide to Data Analysis
Julie Pallant

Praise for previous editions:

'I just wanted to say how much I value Julie Pallant's SPSS Survival Manual. It's quite the best text in SPSS I've encountered and I recommend it to anyone who's listening!'
- Professor Carolyn Hicks, Birmingham University, UK

'There are several SPSS manuals published and this one really does 'do what it says on the tin' ... Whether you are a beginner doing your BSc or struggling with your PhD research (or beyond!), I wholeheartedly recommend this book.'
- British Journal of Occupational Therapy, UK

Praise for the new edition:

'An excellent introduction to using SPSS for data analysis ... It provides a self-contained resource itself, with more than simply (detailed and clear) step-by-step descriptions of statistical procedures in SPSS. There is also a wealth of tips and advice, and for each statistical technique a brief, but consistently reliable, explanation is provided.'
- Associate Professor George Dunbar, Department of Psychology, University of Warwick, UK

In this fully revised edition of her bestselling text, Julie Pallant guides you through the entire research process, helping you choose the right data analysis technique for your project. From the formulation of research questions, to the design of the study and analysis of data, to reporting the results, Julie discusses basic and advanced statistical techniques. She outlines each technique clearly, with step-by-step procedures for performing the analysis, a detailed guide to interpreting SPSS output and an example of how to present the results in a report.

For both beginners and experienced SPSS users in psychology, sociology, health sciences, medicine, education, business and related disciplines, the *SPSS Survival Manual* is an essential guide. Illustrated with screen grabs, examples of output and tips, it is supported by a website with sample data and guidelines on report writing.

In this third edition all chapters have been updated to accommodate changes to SPSS procedures, screens and output in version 15. A new flowchart is included for SPSS procedures, and factor analysis procedures have been streamlined. It also includes more examples and material on syntax. Additional data files are available on the books's supporting website.

Contents: Preface – Data files and website – Introduction and overview – **Part one: Getting started** - Designing a study – Preparing a codebook – Getting to know SPSS – **Part two: Preparing the data file** - Creating a data file and entering data – Screening and cleaning the data – **Part three: Preliminary analyses** – Descriptive statistics – Using graphs to describe and explore the data – Manipulating the data – Checking the reliability of a scale – Choosing the right statistic – **Part four: Statistical techniques to explore relationships among variables** – Correlation – Partial correlation – Multiple regression – Logistic regression – Factor analysis – **Part five: Statistical techniques to compare groups** – Non-parametric statistics – T-tests – One-way analysis of variance – Two-way between-groups ANOVA – Mixed between-within subjects analysis of variance – Multivariate analysis of variance – Analysis of covariance – Appendix: Details of data files – Recommended reading – References – Index

2007 352pp
ISBN: 978-0-335-22366-4 Paperback